CASE STUDIES IN PHYSIOLOGY

CASE STUDIES IN PHYSIOLOGY

Edited by
ROBERT M. BERNE, M.D., D.Sc. (Hon.)
Professor of Physiology, Emeritus
Department of Physiology
University of Virginia Health Sciences Center
Charlottesville, Virginia

MATTHEW N. LEVY, M.D.
Chief of Investigative Medicine, Mount Sinai Medical Center
Professor Emeritus of Physiology and Biophysics and of Biomedical Engineering
Case Western Reserve University
Cleveland, Ohio

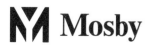 Mosby

St. Louis Baltimore Berlin Boston Carlsbad Chicago London Madrid
Naples New York Philadelphia Sydney Tokyo Toronto

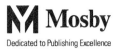
Mosby

Dedicated to Publishing Excellence

Editor: Robert Farrell
Developmental Editor: Emma D. Underdown
Project Manager: Peggy Fagen
Production Editor: Lisa Nomura

Printed in the United States of America
Mosby—Year Book, Inc.
11830 Westline Industrial Drive,
St. Louis, Missouri 63146

94 95 96 97 98/ 9 8 7 6 5 4 3 2 1

Contributors

ROBERT M. BERNE, MD
Professor of Physiology, Emeritus
Department of Physiology
University of Virginia Health Sciences Center
Charlottesville, Virginia
Section V The Cardiovascular System

SAUL M. GENUTH, MD
Professor, Department of Medicine
School of Medicine
Case Western Reserve University
Cleveland, Ohio
Section IX The Endocrine System

BRUCE M. KOEPPEN, MD, PhD
Professor
Department of Medicine and Physiology
University of Connecticut Health Center
Farmington, Connecticut
Section VII The Kidney

HOWARD C. KUTCHAI, PhD
Professor, Department of Physiology
University of Virginia Health Sciences Center
Charlottesville, Virginia
Section I Cellular Physiology
Section VII The Gastrointestinal System

MATTHEW N. LEVY, MD
Chief, Investigative Medicine
Mount Sinai Hospital Medical Center
Cleveland, Ohio
Section V The Cardiovascular System

LAWRENCE MARTIN, MD
Chief, Division of Pulmonary and Critical Care
Medicine
Mount Sinai Medical Center
Cleveland, Ohio
Section VI The Respiratory System

RICHARD A. MURPHY, PhD
Professor, Department of Molecular Physiology
and Biological Physics
University of Virginia School of Medicine
Charlottesville, Virginia
Section III Muscle

OSCAR D. RATNOFF, MD
Professor, School of Medicine
Department of Medicine
Case Western Reserve University
Cleveland, Ohio
Section IV Blood

BRUCE A. STANTON, PhD
Professor, Department of Physiology
Dartmouth College Medical School
Hanover, New Hampshire
Section VIII The Kidney

WILLIAM D. WILLIS, JR., MD, PhD
Asbel Smith Professor and Chairman
Department of Anatomy and Neurosciences
The University of Texas Medical Branch at
Galveston
Galveston, Texas
Section II The Nervous System

Preface

The purposes of this book are to use case histories as a vehicle for reviewing various important physiologic principles, to illustrate how physiology constitutes the basis of medicine, and to indicate how medicine is essentially abnormal physiology. The use of clinical cases makes basic physiology more relevant, especially to the medical student, for whom this book is mainly designed. The questions and answers generally deal with physiologic concepts and principles. All of the questions raised about each case are answered in the back of the book, some in great detail. In addition, references are cited to appropriate pages in the third edition of *Physiology* (edited by Berne and Levy) for a consideration of the physiologic mechanisms that relate to the questions posed.

We hope that this companion book to *Physiology*, third edition, will be helpful to students of this discipline. Also, we welcome criticism and suggestions from the readers, so that future printings and editions can be improved.

Robert M. Berne
Matthew N. Levy

Contents

SECTION VI
THE RESPIRATORY SYSTEM
Lawrence E. Martin

SECTION VII
THE GASTROINTESTINAL SYSTEM
Howard C. Kutchai

SECTION VIII
THE KIDNEY
Bruce A. Stanton
Bruce M. Koeppen

SECTION IX
THE ENDOCRINE SYSTEM
Saul M. Genuth

SECTION X
Answers to Case Study Questions

CELLULAR PHYSIOLOGY

Howard C. Kutchai

CHAPTER 1

Cellular Membranes and Transmembrane Transport of Solutes and Water

Hereditary Spherocytosis

A 20-year-old woman suffers from anemia and occasional jaundice. A thorough review of her medical records reveals that over the past 10 years she has had episodes of more severe anemia, usually after periods of febrile illness. The patient has a markedly enlarged spleen. Microscopic examination of the patient's blood showed a large number of microspherocytes (red blood cells [RBCs] that are round and somewhat smaller than erythrocytes). The osmotic fragility (measured by putting RBCs in hypotonic solutions) was much greater than that of RBCs from healthy individuals. When the patient's erythrocytes were incubated in a buffer solution at 37° C under sterile conditions, the fraction of the RBCs that were hemolyzed was much larger than the hemolyzed fraction from a healthy individual. This "autohemolysis" could be greatly diminished by including glucose and adenosine triphosphate (ATP) in the RBC incubation solution. RBCs from fresh blood had a normal content of Na^+ and K^+. The permeabilities of the patient's erythrocyte membranes to Na^+ and K^+ were found to be about three times normal. The level of Na^+, K^+-ATPase in the patient's RBC membranes was also about three times the level in RBCs from healthy individuals. The average life span of the patient's erythrocytes was well below the normal life span. When an aliquot of the patient's RBCs was labeled and injected intravenously into a healthy individual, the patient's RBCs had a markedly reduced survival time compared with normal RBCs. When labeled RBCs from a healthy individual were infused into the patient, the survival time of the normal RBCs was comparable with their survival time in the donor. The patient's spleen was removed, and after the splenectomy, the patient's anemia was largely ameliorated.

1. Why should the patient's erythrocytes have a greater osmotic fragility than RBCs from healthy individuals?

2. Why might the patient's RBCs "autohemolyze" more rapidly than normal erythrocytes when they are incubated at 37° C under sterile conditions?

3. Why should including glucose and ATP in the incubation mixture diminish the extent of autohemolysis?

4. Why should the patient's RBCs have a reduced life span? What might the spleen have to do with this?

5. What is proved by the observations that the patient's RBCs have a reduced life span in the circulation of a healthy individual and that the RBCs of a healthy individual have a normal life span in the patient's circulation?

6. Why might the patient have more severe episodes of anemia following febrile illnesses?

7. Why should splenectomy largely correct the patient's anemia?

CHAPTER 2

Ionic Equilibria and Resting Membrane Potentials

Primary Hyperkalemic Periodic Paralysis

A 10-year-old boy has sporadic attacks of muscle paralysis. The patient has four brothers, all of whom have suffered similar symptoms. The onset of these attacks is characterized by pain associated with contractures of the affected muscles. Later in the attack those muscles may become paralyzed and more flaccid. Episodes of pain and contracture frequently occur without subsequent paralysis. Analysis of blood samples taken during an attack indicates that the patient is hyperkalemic. Plasma K^+ levels are normal when the patient is not having an attack. Biopsies of the patient's muscle show a significantly diminished level of intracellular K^+ (83 mmol/kg wet tissue) compared with control muscle (95 mmol/kg wet tissue). Basal tissue activity of Na^+, K^+-ATPase is normal. Paralytic attacks are accompanied by diuresis with increased K^+ excretion. Electrophysiologic studies of the patient show that during an attack the excitability and conduction times of motor neurons are normal, as is the function of the neuromuscular junction. Microelectrode studies show that during an attack the magnitude of the resting membrane potential of skeletal muscle cells is diminished compared with control muscle fibers. Electromyography shows that early in an attack the muscle contractures are associated with spontaneous action potentials in the affected muscle fibers. Later, during the paralytic phase of an attack, muscle cells become electrically inexcitable—the muscle cells do not respond electrically to stimulation of the motor axons that innervate them. A paralytic attack can be relieved by treating the patient with an insulin injection. Long-term administration of the β_2-agonist salbutamol dramatically diminishes the occurrence of episodes of both contractures and subsequent paralytic attacks.

1. What might account for the patient being hyperkalemic during an attack, while the potassium concentration in his skeletal muscle cells is diminished? What types of alterations of basic cellular processes might underlie this situation?

2. What explains the observation that the magnitude of the resting membrane potentials of the patient's skeletal muscle fibers is diminished during an attack?

3. Does the diminished resting membrane potential have anything to do with the spontaneous action potentials and contractures that occur early in an attack, before paralysis sets in?

4. How might the diminished resting membrane potential contribute to the paralytic phase of an attack, in which muscle cells are electrically inexcitable?

5. How might insulin terminate a paralytic attack?

6. How might long-term administration of salbutamol diminish the occurrence of attacks of contractures and paralysis?

CHAPTER 3

Generation and Conduction of Action Potentials

Poisoning with Saxitoxin

A 30-year-old woman is brought into the emergency room. The patient had been dining in a local restaurant, and while eating dessert she noted the following symptoms. Initially there was a tingling sensation that affected the mouth and lips, but then it spread to the face and neck. Then the tingling spread down the arms and legs to the fingers and toes.

At the hospital the patient reports numbness of the areas that previously tingled and difficulty walking in a coordinated fashion. The patient is asked to describe the meal she has just eaten and states that she had shrimp cocktail as an appetizer, followed by salad, steak with a baked potato and green beans, and apple pie and coffee for dessert. The patient has no history of allergic response to shellfish. Her superficial reflexes are almost absent, and her deep reflexes are markedly hypoactive. An extracellular electrode is placed on the patient's ulnar nerve. Then the palmar surface of the patient's little finger is scraped with the physician's fingernail in a way that should be painful to the patient. The patient cannot feel this stimulus, and no action potentials are detected in the ulnar nerve. When an intracellular microelectrode is placed on a sensory nerve fiber in the ulnar nerve, the resting membrane potential is found to be near -70 mV (normal). When an action potential is evoked by repeated vigorous scraping of the skin of the little finger as described earlier, the action potential is slower to rise and of shorter height than expected from measurements in normal individuals. The duration of the action potential is normal.

1. What can be concluded from the failure of vigorous scraping of the skin of the little finger to elicit action potentials in the ulnar nerve?

2. What can be concluded from the gross neurologic symptoms and findings taken together?

3. What can be concluded from the finding that the resting membrane potential in the sensory fibers in the ulnar nerve is near normal?

4. What might explain the finding that the action potential in the sensory fiber in the ulnar nerve is slow to rise and of smaller height than normal?

5. Why is the action potential in the sensory fiber of normal duration?

6. What may be the cause of this patient's difficulties?

7. How should this patient's care be managed, and what is her prognosis?

CHAPTER 4

Synaptic Transmission

Weakness and IgG

A 43-year-old man presents symptoms that include weakness of the lower limbs. The patient complains of difficulty in climbing stairs. On examination he has diminished muscle stretch reflexes. There is a transient increase in muscle power after maximal exercise. Electromyographic (EMG) studies of this patient reveal a diminished amplitude of compound muscle action potentials. The compound muscle action potential is increased by over 200% in amplitude after vigorous exercise of the muscle studied. Single fiber muscle action potentials show significant block (i.e., an action potential in the motor neuron fails to elicit an action potential in the muscle).

After purified IgG from this patient was injected intravenously into a mouse, the mouse displayed signs similar to those of the patient. Studies of the neuromuscular junctions of the mouse's diaphragm revealed that endplate potentials recorded by microelectrodes in the muscle were greatly reduced. The frequency of miniature endplate potentials (mEPPs) in the IgG-injected mouse was similar to the mEPP frequency in diaphragms from control mice. However, when the diaphragms were bathed in elevated K^+ (17.5 mM), the mEPP frequency in the diaphragms from control mice increased dramatically, in contrast to a very slight increase in mEPP frequency in diaphragms from IgG-injected mice. When diaphragms were treated with low doses of a calcium ionophore, the frequency of mEPPs greatly increased (this response was the same in diaphragms from IgG-treated mice and from control mice).

Adrenal chromaffin cells release their chromaffin granule contents by exocytosis, by a process that resembles events in presynaptic nerve terminals. (Chromaffin cells can be patch clamped.) When bovine adrenal chromaffin cells were treated with IgG from the patient, the whole-cell Ca^{++} current elicited by depolarization of the cells decreased dramatically to 0 mV (compared with control cells not treated with IgG). When individual Ca^{++} channels were studied by patch clamp, their properties were not altered by the treatment with the patient's IgG.

The patient was subjected to the following separate therapeutic interventions: (1) plasmapheresis, (2) immunosuppressive therapy, and (3) treatment with 4-aminopyridine (which blocks voltage-dependent K^+ channels). Each of these interventions improved the patient's condition.

1. Why might depolarization-induced Ca^{++} currents in adrenal chromaffin cells be diminished by treating the cells with IgG from the patient?

2. What can you conclude from the observation that single Ca^{++} channels were not affected by the patient's IgG?

3. What can you conclude from the observations that the frequency of mEPPs in diaphragms of control and IgG-injected mice was similar, but that the response to treating the preparation with elevated K^+ was so different (i.e., the frequency of mEPPs increased much more in the diaphragms of control mice)?

4. What can you conclude from the observation that the increase in frequency of mEPPs was similar in diaphragms from control and IgG-injected mice in response to treatment with the calcium ionophore?

5. Why are normal EPPs (evoked by motor neuron stimulation) reduced in size in diaphragms from IgG-injected mice compared with those from control mice?

6. Why should "blocking" be observed in single-fiber EMG studies of the patient's muscles?

7. Why should the amplitude of the compound muscle action potential be reduced in response to voluntary contractions of a muscle (compared with a normal individual)?

8. Why should vigorous exercise of the involved muscle result in a marked increase in the amplitude of the compound muscle action potential?

9. Why should muscular weakness be confined to the patient's lower limbs?

CHAPTER 5

Membrane Receptors, Second Messengers, and Signal Transduction Pathways

Cholera

A 32-year-old woman is brought, almost comatose, into a clinic in Bangladesh during the monsoon season. She has severe diarrhea and is producing watery stool at the rate of nearly 1 L/hr. Her skin appears shriveled, and when a fold of skin is pinched, it remains so for several minutes. Microscopic examination of the patient's stool reveals the presence of a large number of *Vibrio cholerae* bacteria. The patient cannot drink, so intravenous isotonic NaCl is administered. When the patient is fully conscious, she is given a rehydration solution to drink. This oral rehydration solution contains glucose, NaCl, KCl, and $NaHCO_3$. After about 5 days the patient had recovered sufficiently to leave the hospital.

1. What is the pathophysiologic mechanism of the patient's diarrhea?

2. How do intravenous fluids improve the patient's condition?

3. What is the rationale for administering the oral rehydration solution to the patient?

4. Why does the patient recover in about 5 days?

THE NERVOUS SYSTEM

William D. Willis, Jr.

CHAPTER 6

The Nervous System and Its Components

Hydrocephalus

A 3-month-old infant was admitted to the pediatrics ward because of failure to thrive and a large head. The infant stayed quietly in bed most of the day. The circumference of the head was 45 cm (normal value for this age is about 40 cm). The fontanelles protruded, and the cranial sutures were separated. The skull could be transilluminated with a flashlight. Magnetic resonance imaging showed enlarged lateral, third, and fourth ventricles. The closure of the vertebrae was defective in the lower back (spina bifida). Treatment was surgical implantation of a catheter into the lateral ventricle with drainage into the peritoneum.

1. Why are the ventricles dilated in this infant?

2. Is this a communicating or noncommunicating type of hydrocephalus?

3. What might cause this type of hydrocephalus in an infant?

4. What cerebrospinal fluid pressure would you expect in the ventricles? What is the normal level in infants?

5. In cases like this, what tends to happen to the following intracranial fluid volumes: cerebrospinal fluid, brain, and blood?

6. How can this condition affect mental function as the infant grows? What are some potential problems associated with the surgical shunt procedure?

7. Can anything similar to this happen in adults?

8. What are some of the possible complications of the associated spina bifida in this infant?

CHAPTER 7

The Peripheral Nervous System

Gunshot Wound

An 18-year-old high school senior was shot in the left thigh as he left school. On examination in the hospital emergency room, he was found to have weakness of his ankle dorsiflexors, evertors, and invertors, toe flexors, and hamstring muscles. He had sensory loss over the lateral aspect of the leg, the dorsal surface of the foot, and the sole of the foot. The sciatic nerve was exposed surgically and found to be severed. A nerve graft was used to repair the interruption. At a subsequent visit to his physician several weeks later, the weakness was present, and the muscle supplied by the sciatic nerve showed marked atrophy. Electromyography in several of these muscles revealed an absence of motor unit discharges, but frequent fibrillations. Over the next year, there was progressive proximal to distal recovery of some motor function, but there was some residual weakness.

1. What caused the weakness in the left lower extremity?

2. What caused the sensory loss?

3. Would there also be autonomic changes in the left leg?

4. Why did the muscles supplied by the sciatic nerve undergo atrophy?

5. Why were there no motor unit potentials several weeks after the injury? Why were there fibrillations at this time? How can fibrillations be distinguished from motor unit potentials by electromyography?

6. What accounts for the progressive proximal to distal recovery in motor function?

7. Why is recovery incomplete?

8. Would there be sensory recovery as well?

9. Where are the cellular materials made that are needed for the regeneration of motor axons? Sensory axons?

10. How are these materials transferred along the growing axons?

CHAPTER 8

The Somatosensory System

Case 1: Sensory Loss After Knife Wound

A 23-year-old woman was brought by an ambulance to the emergency room. She had been in a fight and had been stabbed in the back at a midthoracic level with a butcher knife. A sensory examination revealed a loss of vibratory sense in the right ankle and loss of position sense in the great toe of the right foot. Pain and temperature sensation on the left side was lost below the umbilicus. She was unable to move her right lower extremity, and stretch reflexes were absent in that limb. One month later the sensory deficits were still present. At this time the reflexes in the right lower extremity were hyperactive, and an extensor plantar response (sign of Babinski) was present on the right. However, her right limb was still weak. Her condition did not change substantially at follow-up examinations over the next several years.

1. What part of the nervous system was damaged by the knife wound?

2. What was the segmental level of the nervous system lesion? Of the back wound?

3. Interruption of what central nervous system pathway explains the loss of pain and temperature sensations on the left side?

4. Interruption of what central nervous system pathways explains the loss of vibratory and position sense in the right leg?

5. Why was touch not lost? Why was vibratory or position sense on the lower trunk not lost?

6. What sense organs signal vibratory and position sense?

7. Why was the right lower extremity paralyzed?

8. Why were the stretch reflexes absent at first and then later hyperactive?

9. Why did a sign of Babinski appear?

10. Why was recovery of function so poor?

Case 2: Colon Cancer

A 75-year-old man developed cancer of the colon. The cancer resulted in severe pain, because of both visceral pain and metastases to bone of the vertebral column. Morphine controlled the pain initially, but eventually the pain became so severe that the required high doses of morphine interfered with the ability of the patient to think clearly. Several options were considered to improve the quality of the patient's life during his terminal period: 1) installation of a patient-controlled epidural morphine pump; 2) bilateral cordotomies; and 3) deep brain stimulation.

1. Why was morphine able to control the cancer pain initially? That is, where and how does morphine act when given systemically to control pain?

2. How would epidural infusion of morphine be able to control the pain of colon cancer? What is the advantage of allowing a patient to control a morphine pump?

3. What can be done if an inadvertent overdose of morphine leads to respiratory arrest?

4. What are the advantages and disadvantages of anterolateral cordotomy?

5. What would be a suitable target for deep brain stimulation to control cancer pain?

CHAPTER 9

The Visual System

Acromegaly with Visual Field Defect

A 35-year-old man comes to his physician because of changes in his appearance. His hands and feet have been growing, and his brow and chin are also becoming larger. On examination the patient did not see the fingers of the examiner when they were moved in either superior temporal visual field. Detailed visual field examination by an ophthalmologist revealed a visual field defect in both temporal fields, but the defect was more complete in the superior rather than in the inferior quadrants. The patient was referred to a neurosurgeon for treatment.

    1.   What is the most likely cause of the changes in the patient's appearance?

    2.   What hormone is being secreted in excess?

    3.   What type of visual field defect did the patient have?

    4.   What caused the visual field defect? Why was the defect more complete in the superior rather than in the inferior temporal quadrants?

CHAPTER 10

The Auditory and Vestibular Systems

Acoustic Neurinoma

A 47-year-old man saw his family physician because of headaches and an unsteady gait. The patient had a long history of difficulties with hearing in his right ear. Fourteen years previously, he experienced a ringing in that ear, but since then he had become progressively more deaf on the right side. In addition, his gait became unsteady, and he tended to fall toward the right. Five years ago, he developed numbness on the right side of his face, and this has since spread to include the right half of the tongue. A year ago, he developed pain in the occipital area, and he sometimes became nauseated. The right side of his face became weak, and it was observed that his right eye constantly remained open. The neurologic examination revealed the following abnormalities. The right eyelid was open and seldom blinked, and the right side of the face was immobile. The right corneal reflex was absent. Taste was lost on the right side of the tongue. The right eye could not be deviated to the right beyond the midline. Nystagmus appeared when the patient moved his eyes horizontally. Sensation was lost on right side of the face. When the patient was asked to say "ah," the soft palate deviated to the left. Examination of the eyes with an ophthalmoscope revealed papilledema bilaterally. The patient walked with a wide stance, and he lurched to the right. His right arm showed incoordination in the finger-to-nose test. An audiogram showed a complete hearing loss for the right ear, and a caloric test was completely negative on the right. Eighth nerve function was normal for the left ear. In the Weber test, sound was localized to the left ear; the Rinne test was normal for the left ear, but no sound was heard on the right. The patient was referred to a neurosurgeon for removal of an acoustic neurinoma.

1. What cranial nerves were affected in this patient?

2. What accounts for the headaches, papilledema, and nausea?

3. Is the type of deafness conductive or sensorineural?

4. Explain the negative caloric test on the right.

5. Explain the loss of taste on the right side of the tongue.

6. Explain the loss of sensation on the right side of the face.

7. Account for the lurching gait and the ataxia of the right arm.

CHAPTER 11

The Chemical Senses

Meningioma

A 52-year-old woman noticed a gradual loss of vision in both eyes, and she experienced progressively severe headaches. A careful examination by her physician revealed that her right optic disc was pale and that she had a central scotoma on the right side. The margin of the left optic disc was blurred, the central veins of the retina were dilated, and the optic disc protruded by 2 diopters from the surface of the retina. Some hemorrhages and exudates were noted in the retina around the optic disc. On further testing the patient could not recognize odors introduced into her right nostril, but her sense of smell was intact on the left.

1. Why was the patient unable to recognize odors in the right nostril?

2. What is a possible cause for this malfunction?

3. What caused the central scotoma in the right eye?

4. What is wrong with the left eye? What has caused this?

5. Can anything be done for the patient? What residual deficits are likely after successful treatment?

CHAPTER 12

Spinal Organization of Motor Function

Spinal Cord Injury

A 19-year-old man hyperextended his neck in a car accident. He lost consciousness for a short time, and when he awoke he could not move any of his limbs, nor could he feel any sensations in his trunk or limbs. After a month he could move his shoulders to some extent, but otherwise, all four extremities remained paralyzed. At this time he developed increased muscle tone and hyperactive stretch reflexes in both arms and legs. Also, when either foot was sharply dorsiflexed, sustained clonus of the ankle occurred. Signs of Babinski could readily be elicited bilaterally. Stimulation of one foot caused withdrawal of that foot and also flexion of the other leg. He had to be catheterized to allow drainage of the urinary bladder.

1. At what level was the spinal cord functionally transected?

2. Why was the patient unable to move his extremities?

3. Why was all sensation lost in the trunk and extremities?

4. Would the phasic or the tonic stretch reflexes be more affected? What causes clonus?

5. Why do flexion reflexes become more active?

6. How did urinary bladder function change?

CHAPTER 13

Descending Pathways Involved in Motor Control

Hemiparesis

A 58-year-old woman, who was known to be hypertensive, was brought to the hospital one morning. She awoke paralyzed on the right side and unable to talk. Her blood pressure was 230/120. Her heartbeat was irregular, and eyegrounds showed narrowing of the arteries, hemorrhages, and exudates. She could not move her right arm and leg voluntarily. When asked to move her right arm, she picked it up with the left one. When she tried to smile, the facial muscles on the left side of her face contracted, but those on the right side did not. However, she could furrow her brow bilaterally and close both eyes tightly. The phasic stretch reflexes were increased in the right extremities, and the sign of Babinski was present on the right side. Sensory tests were difficult to perform because of the speech problem.

1. What problem was responsible for the neurologic deficits?

2. What part of the central nervous system did the lesion affect? On which side?

3. What motor pathways were interrupted? Why could the patient still furrow her brow and close her eyes?

4. What kind of speech problem did she have?

5. What sensory deficits might she have, if these could be tested?

CHAPTER 14

Motor Control by the Cerebral Cortex, Cerebellum, and Basal Ganglia

Case 1: Multiple Sclerosis

A 26-year-old woman is hospitalized because of several neurologic problems. When she was 21, she had a transient episode of blindness. She could not see objects in the center of the visual field of her left eye. At 23, she developed a motor problem in her hands, but she recovered in a few weeks. Her present illness is characterized by ataxia of gait, a tendency to fall, and nystagmus. Examination revealed that her left optic nerve was much paler than her right optic nerve. She had an intention tremor in her arms when she was asked to touch her nose, and she had difficulty in making alternating pronation and supination movements of her arms.

1. Does the patient have a single, discrete lesion of her central nervous system? What caused her earlier central scotoma?

2. Her motor problems can be ascribed to damage to what structure?

3. If the phasic stretch reflexes in her lower extremities are tested, what are their likely characteristics?

Case 2: Parkinson's Disease

A 49-year-old man sees his physician to renew his prescription. As he sits in the waiting room, he is observed to have a tremor in his hands and fingers. His face is unexpressive, and he makes few movements. When he is invited to enter the physician's office, he has difficulty in standing up. He walks slowly into the office, and his arms do not swing appreciably. When he talks to the physician, his speech is monotonous, but he shows no intellectual deficit.

1. In what ways does this man's tremor differ from that of the patient in the previous case?

2. Why are the movements so few and slow? Are the phasic stretch reflexes altered?

3. What part of the nervous system is involved in this disease?

CHAPTER 15

The Autonomic Nervous System and Its Central Control

Horner's Syndrome

A 62-year-old man suddenly developed an ataxic gait, and he tended to fall to the right. His right arm and leg became clumsy, and he became hoarse. When he was asked to stand with his feet together, he tended to fall to the right, whether his eyes were open or closed. The right eyelid drooped, and the right pupil was distinctly smaller than the left. He did not sweat on the right side of the face. Pain and temperature sensations were decreased on the right side of the face and over the left side of the body and left limbs.

1. Where in the central nervous system was the lesion? What was the cause of the somatic sensory deficits?

2. What was the cause of the autonomic changes in the right eye and face?

3. What was the motor disorder affecting gait? Why did the patient become hoarse?

CHAPTER 16

The Cerebral Cortex and Higher Functions of the Nervous System

Case 1: Narcolepsy

A 35-year-old man is admitted to the hospital because he was injured in a car accident. He was driving home after work and fell asleep at the wheel. He has had three such accidents in the past year. He also falls asleep regularly at work, at the dinner table, at church, and in fact, anywhere. He reports other peculiar symptoms. When he becomes excited or enraged, he suddenly becomes weak and falls. At night he often has bizarre, terrifying dreams. During these dreams he feels as if he were paralyzed. His diagnosis is narcolepsy, and a stimulant drug is prescribed.

1. Which sleep state do the symptoms of narcolepsy resemble?

2. What would the electroencephalogram look like during the sleep of a narcoleptic?

3. Why would a stimulant drug be useful in the treatment of narcolepsy?

Case 2: Epilepsy

A 28-year-old man is brought to the hospital by the police. He was found lying in the gutter, unconscious and with his clothing soaked with mud, blood, and urine. He has a cut over his eyebrow, and his limbs are bruised. He does not remember falling, but he related that this kind of experience has occurred to him frequently in the past, ever since he was 11 years old. His recent seizure began with his head and eyes turning toward the right, and these actions were followed by movements of his right hand. After this he fell and hit his head, his body became rigid, he turned blue, and then he started to jerk. Toward the end of his seizure, he urinated. Finally, he relaxed and remained unconscious for about half an hour. On awakening, he remembers having a headache and feeling depressed. His muscles were sore. An electroencephalogram was taken, but it showed only diffuse abnormalities, nothing that would help localize the source of the problem. An anticonvulsant drug was prescribed, and he was admitted for observation of possible sequelae of the head injury.

1. What type of epilepsy did the patient have?

2. What do the movements preceding the generalized seizure signify?

3. What would the electroencephalogram have been like during the seizure?

4. What might be the neurophysiologic basis for a seizure state?

MUSCLE

Richard A. Murphy

CHAPTER 17

Contractile Mechanism of Muscle Cells

Delayed Onset of Muscle Soreness

The fitness of a group of individuals of various ages and both genders was assessed in a step test. The test consisted of stepping up and down 18 inches (46 cm) 15 times per minute, for 20 minutes. The stepping pattern produced shortening of the right quadriceps muscle during the step up. The descent was opposed by contraction of the left quadriceps muscle that was stretched by the force of gravity. The subjects reported feeling weakness in the left quadriceps muscle. The weakness lasted for approximately 2 hours, and maximum voluntary force development was less than the preexercise value. Percutaneous electrical stimulation of the quadriceps elicited reduced forces. Pain developed in the left quadriceps 8 to 10 hours after the exercise, reached maximal intensity between 24 and 48 hours, and persisted for about a week. This delayed onset of muscular soreness (DOMS) induced by exercise was marked in activities that imposed negative work on the muscle; such activities include descending stairs. The magnitude of the soreness was unrelated to the overall fitness of the individuals, but specific training for this step test prevented soreness in subsequent tests.

Evidence of muscle cell injury included an increase in serum levels of soluble proteins, such as creatine kinase and myoglobin. The time course was similar to that of the soreness. Myofibrillar disorganization and sarcolemmal disruption could be observed in biopsy samples from only the left quadriceps.

1. Have you experienced DOMS? What are the circumstances that lead to DOMS and increase its severity?

2. Why was DOMS experienced in only the left quadriceps muscle in this fairly moderate exercise?

3. Is an impaired adenosine triphosphate (ATP) supply or synthetic capacity a reasonable explanation for the fatigue of the left quadriceps muscle?

4. One hypothesis for the etiology of DOMS is that increased metabolism results in the accumulation of toxic waste products. Can this explain the soreness?

5. Exercise can raise the temperature of an active muscle by 5° C or more. Is heat injury a plausible explanation for DOMS?

6. Are there clinical signs of muscle cell injury?

7. What is a plausible mechanism for injury of muscle cells or their tendons?

8. What does DOMS suggest about the adaptability of muscle fibers to use?

9. Pain is usually regarded (teleologically) as a signal to protect the organism from injury. Is this a rational explanation for DOMS?

10. What might be responsible for the slow development of stiffness and soreness?

CHAPTER 18

Skeletal Muscle Physiology

Case 1: Cardiomyoplasty for Ventricular Aneurysm

In a currently experimental treatment, a patient with a left ventricular aneurysm underwent an operation in which the aneurysm was surgically removed. To help the weakened heart, the left latissimus dorsi (skeletal) muscle was dissected free from its normal location in the lower back where it inserts on the humerus and is active in all pulling movements. Maintaining its major neurovascular connections (pedicle), the muscle was moved into the thoracic cavity and wrapped around the heart in an orientation that would compress the left ventricle on contraction of the latissimus dorsi. A "cardiomyostimulator" was implanted to electrically stimulate the latissimus dorsi via its motor nerves in synchrony with the heartbeat. After a conditioning and training period of several weeks, the functional capacity of the patient to undertake modest activity was improved by the operation (termed dynamic cardiomyoplasty).

1. Is the latissimus dorsi a suitable substitute for cardiac muscle if one assumes that the formidable technical problems could be overcome?

2. Could a standard cardiac pacemaker be used to drive the latissimus dorsi?

3. How can the problem of fatigue be solved?

4. What vascular adaptations would be required in the latissimus dorsi?

5. Before the operation the sarcomere length of the latissimus dorsi would be near the optimal for force generation, or around 2.2 μm at rest. How might this change after surgery?

6. The skeleton normally prevents significant shortening of skeletal muscle cells. How can the latissimus dorsi generate large forces if there are no skeletal restraints to shortening?

7. In the process of establishing an adequate vascular system there is considerable proliferation and growth of vascular smooth muscle cells in the latissimus dorsi. Why doesn't this occur in the myocardium with proliferation and replacement of cardiac muscle cells to repair the damage?

8. Heart failure is fairly common. Is cardiomyoplasty likely to supersede cardiac transplants as a surgical therapy?

9. Why wouldn't pulling efforts with the left arm postoperatively lead to compression of the heart by the latissimus dorsi?

10. The pacemaker should activate the afferent sensory nerve fibers as well as the motor nerve fibers. What are the potential results?

Case 2: Duchenne Muscular Dystrophy

Duchenne muscular dystrophy is a devastating, progressive disease that occurs in boys; it is characterized by the progressive necrosis of skeletal muscle fibers and death at an average age of 16, usually from respiratory failure. It is the second most common genetic disorder in humans, and there is no specific treatment. The course of the disease includes slow muscular development, progressive weakness, and frequent contractures. The disease is usually recognized at ages 2 to 5, and the child is usually confined to a wheelchair by age 12. Laboratory observations show highly elevated serum concentrations of creatine kinase and other soluble sarcoplasmic enzymes. Both fast and slow muscle fibers are affected by fiber necrosis and phagocytosis, balanced by marked regeneration of cells in the early stages of the disease. The fibers resemble fetal muscles, in terms of their isoenzyme patterns, with marked dedifferentiation. Fiber death and replacement by fat and connective tissue gradually predominate. DNA analysis reveals that the disease is caused by the deficiency of a gene on the X chromosome. The product of the gene is a cytoskeletal protein called dystrophin that forms a network adjacent to the sarcolemma. Dystrophin is a very large protein (426 kDa). It is a minor constituent of muscle and links sarcomeres to the sarcolemma via association with a glycoprotein inserted into the membrane.

1. Diseases affecting striated muscle cells are uncommon but are devastating and characteristically lethal. Why?

2. What is the significance of the elevated serum creatine kinase level?

3. Is elevated serum creatine kinase diagnostic for muscular dystrophy?

4. Some muscles are more affected than others. In fact, the muscles of the calves exhibit a characteristic hypertrophy, whereas the muscles of the upper legs are weakened. What factors may influence differential responses in a patient whose skeletal muscle cells lack a functional dystrophin gene?

5. Why is Duchenne muscular dystrophy progressive even though the genetic defect is present from conception?

6. Why don't girls develop Duchenne muscular dystrophy?

7. Exercise is a major component of the clinical management of Duchenne muscular dystrophy. What is the rationale?

8. Would the introduction of a functional allele of the dystrophin gene in the affected cells be a potential treatment that could cure the disease?

Case 3: Malignant Hyperthermia

A patient received succinylcholine (muscle relaxant) and halothane (general anesthetic) for routine gall-bladder surgery. Instead of the expected muscle relaxation, massive fasciculations (spontaneous motor unit contractions) were followed by rigidity of muscles (contracture characterized by hard muscles and unmovable joints). Tachycardia developed along with hypertension. A marked increase in respiration was driven by elevated arterial carbon dioxide tension. The core body temperature then began to rise rapidly (up to 44° C), reflecting increased metabolism of skeletal muscle. Hyperthermia and cardiac arrhythmias led to left ventricular failure and resulted in acute pulmonary edema. Increased muscle metabolism decreased blood oxygen and blood pH. The acidosis is of both metabolic (increased serum lactate) and respiratory (increased blood carbon dioxide) origin. Serum concentrations of soluble muscle proteins, such as creatine kinase, lactate dehydrogenase, and myoglobin, increased markedly.

The symptoms led to a diagnosis of malignant hyperthermia, and the patient was treated with dantrolene, a drug that blocks release of Ca^{++} from the sarcoplasmic reticulum. The crisis passed, but severe muscle pain with swelling lasted for many days. Muscle weakness and wasting occurred for some weeks. Subsequent investigation showed that the patient had a number of relatives who had experienced malignant hyperthermia during anesthesia or died with similar symptoms without an obvious cause.

1. Fasciculation and muscular rigidity reflect pathologic contractions of skeletal muscle cells. What would induce this at the cellular level?

2. What are the clinical signs of a massive increase in metabolism?

3. What is the probable tissue source of the increased metabolism?

4. What metabolic pathways are involved in the increase in metabolism?

5. Will muscle ATP levels be maintained?

6. Elevated cell Ca^{++} is typically associated with cell death. What are potential causes of pathologically elevated cell Ca^{++} and subsequent cell death?

7. What is the evidence for a defective membrane component in the skeletal muscle of patients experiencing malignant hyperthermia?

CHAPTER 19

Smooth Muscle

Case 1: Esophageal Reflux

A 30-year-old man went to see his physician because of repeated episodes of substernal burning pain, which usually occurred shortly after eating. Because an antacid like Rolaids usually relieved the discomfort, he dismissed the problem as heartburn. However, the persistence of his symptoms and his family history of heart disease convinced him to get a checkup. Results of his physical examination were normal, and findings from the electrocardiogram, stress test, and chest x-ray examination were all normal. His physician assured him that his heart was normal and that his symptoms were caused by reflux of acid gastric contents into the esophagus, possibly caused by esophageal sphincter incompetence.

1. What are the physical factors that move materials along hollow organs?

2. What are the physical barriers to gastroesophageal reflux?

3. How might a retrograde pressure gradient be established from the stomach into the esophagus?

4. What are the muscle components of the esophagus and their functions?

5. Is the striated muscle of the esophagus skeletal or cardiac? Why?

6. The movement of a bolus of food down the esophagus is uniform with no major differences between the skeletal, mixed, or smooth muscle regions. How can this be explained, given the striking contrasts in shortening velocity and power output between smooth and skeletal muscle?

7. Tone in the lower esophageal sphincter (the circular layer of the distal 3 to 4 cm of the esophagus) varies, but it is not abolished by denervation and it is not caused by a train of smooth muscle action potentials. Tone persists if the sphincter is dissected and placed in an organ bath in vitro. What mechanisms may be involved in maintaining tone under these conditions?

8. What causes the lower esophageal sphincter to relax as food passes down the esophagus?

9. What would you expect the relative ATP consumption rates of the upper and lower esophageal sphincters to be when they are maintaining comparable levels of tone?

10. Heartburn is often intensified or triggered when an individual bends over or lies down, especially after eating. Explain.

11. Apart from the symptoms described by patients, can you think of some reasonable clinical tests to detect gastroesophageal reflux?

12. Why can some foods or drinks precipitate gastroesophageal reflux and heartburn whereas comparable volumes of others do not?

Case 2: Asthma

A 20-year-old woman with a long history of asthmatic attacks was rushed to the hospital emergency room because of severe respiratory distress. The current asthmatic attack failed to respond to the usual antihistamine drug that was self-administered. When seen by the emergency room physician, the woman was sitting up, obviously anxious, and desperately trying to breathe. She was slightly cyanotic, sweating, wheezing, and had a heart rate of 120 beats/min. She was given oxygen and epinephrine, and her symptoms subsided considerably, although wheezing and crackling sounds were still audible by auscultation, and she was extremely fatigued.

1. What is the physical cause of the dyspnea (difficulty in breathing) and fatigue?

2. What factors might contribute to airway narrowing?

3. What causes the characteristic wheezing with inspiration and expiration?

4. Why is wheezing first observed during expiration at the onset of an asthmatic attack?

5. What are the kinds of stimuli that can influence airway smooth muscle activation?

6. Why is smooth muscle an important component of the airways?

7. List the types of muscle involved in asthmatic attacks.

8. Does fatigue occur in all of the muscles involved in an asthmatic attack?

9. Would a drug that relaxes airway smooth muscle relieve an asthmatic attack if the drug was properly formulated as an inhalant?

10. Would a drug that was effective in reducing airway resistance by relaxing airway smooth muscle decrease pulmonary blood pressure?

11. Why would an asthmatic attack be associated with hyperinflated lungs?

12. In what ways can a drug or physiologic regulator acting on the sarcolemma of an airway smooth muscle bring about relaxation?

Case 3: Childbirth

A 24-year-old woman entered the hospital on the advice of her obstetrician because she was having strong labor pains at shorter and shorter intervals. On admission, physical examination revealed a normal pregnant woman in active labor and with dilation of the cervix of 1 to 2 cm. Shortly thereafter, her membranes ruptured, and she gave birth to a healthy 8-pound boy. Her postpartum course was uneventful.

1. What are the functional roles of smooth muscle in the uterus?

2. What types of patterns of contractile activity characterize the uterus?

3. Is smooth muscle different in men and women?

4. What is the striking difference between smooth muscle in reproductive organs and that in most other tissues?

5. During pregnancy, action potentials do not propagate over long distances in the myometrium, and different areas of the myometrium behave independently. Shortly before delivery the electrical and mechanical activity of the entire myometrium becomes synchronous. What changes in the sarcolemma must occur to explain this change?

6. In what way is the relative absence of gap junctions during pregnancy and their presence at delivery functionally essential?

7. What changes at term might be the signal for the formation of gap junctions in the myometrium?

8. What is the myoplasmic second messenger involved in excitation-contraction coupling in the myometrium?

9. What is the source of the Ca^{++} mobilized in response to action potentials?

10. How does an increase in the myoplasmic Ca^{++} concentration produce contraction in myometrial smooth muscle?

11. Why is force not sustained, and why does the myometrium relax between phasic contractions?

12. Why are uterine contractions much slower than the cardiac contractions?

13. Does the cervical smooth muscle relax in response to propagated action potentials?

14. What factors are responsible for the increase in myometrial mass during pregnancy?

15. What are the stimuli for myometrial smooth muscle growth during pregnancy and for its postpartum reversal?

Case 4: Raynaud's Disease

A 32-year-old woman sees her family physician because of episodes of severe pain in her hands, associated with skin color changes and coldness of the hands. These attacks usually occurred during the winter and after exposure of the hands to cold. The physician precipitated one of these attacks by having the patient put her hands in a basin of cold water. At first the hands turned white, and this was associated with increasing pain of the fingers. Then the hands turned slightly cyanotic, followed rapidly by redness and throbbing discomfort. Gradually the pain disappeared, and the hands returned to normal color. The patient was told that she had Raynaud's disease and that she should avoid exposure of her hands to cold.

1. The ability of any muscle to generate force decreases with shortening below the optimum length for force generation. How can vascular smooth muscle contraction occlude an artery when the blood pressure opposing shortening remains at normal levels?

2. Do the mechanisms that regulate vascular smooth muscle activation precisely match blood flow to that needed to provide oxygen and substrates to the muscles of the fingers?

3. Would cooling affect muscle function in the fingers?

4. Is there anything about smooth muscle that would make it more temperature-sensitive than skeletal muscle?

5. Is an impaired ATP synthetic capacity and a form of rigor mortis a reasonable explanation for cooling-induced vasospasm?

6. Why is Raynaud's disease usually an inconvenience rather than a condition that precipitates ulceration and gangrene?

7. What is responsible for the color(s) of the affected fingers?

8. In what sense is the term *vasospasm* misleading?

9. What is responsible for the bright red color of the affected fingers after an attack?

10. What is the normal response of cutaneous blood vessels in the hand to warming or cooling?

11. What normally mediates the response of the cutaneous blood vessels to temperature?

12. Is it significant that individuals with Raynaud's disease often are susceptible to migraine headaches or angina?

13. What would be the effect of denervation of the cutaneous blood vessels of the hand?

14. Denervated cutaneous blood vessels slowly regain spontaneous tone. Is this attributable to reinnervation by sympathetic fibers?

15. Could vasospasm be caused by a loss of normal inactivation or vasodilator function rather than an enhanced constrictor response?

BLOOD

Oscar D. Ratnoff

CHAPTER 20

Blood Components

Upper Gastrointestinal Bleeding

A 30-year-old man, a middle-management executive, consults his physician in a state of panic because for the last 2 weeks his stools have been intermittently black. Although he had considered himself healthy, he in fact has been aware of daily epigastric discomfort and pain over the last 2 years. His distress occurred at first late in the afternoon and more recently also in the middle of the night, awakening him from sleep. He has been relieving the pain by eating food or by taking Tums, tablets of calcium carbonate, but he has taken no other medications. In the past week, the patient has also noticed that he becomes short of breath (dyspneic) when he climbs a flight of stairs. The patient has been under considerable stress at work, he drinks very few alcoholic beverages, but he is a heavy cigarette smoker.

The physician notes that the patient is exceptionally pale; the pallor is most obvious in the conjunctivae and the nail beds. Except for a resting heart rate of 100 beats/min (a slightly high value) and doubtful tenderness on palpation of the epigastrium, the patient's physical examination is unremarkable. Stool obtained by rectal examination is indeed black, and a guaiac test, performed on the stool to check for blood, is positive.

1. An immediate concern is whether the patient's pallor, dyspnea, and marginally elevated heart rate are related to the presence of blood in the stool. To assess this possibility, what laboratory studies would you order immediately?

2. The patient's hematocrit was 21%, hemoglobin was 6 g/dL, and the red blood cell count was 4 million/μL. What can you deduce from these values?

3. Hypochromic microcytic anemia is commonplace in patients with chronic blood loss and reflects depletion of the iron stores needed for hemoglobin synthesis. If the patient had lost blood in a single brief event (e.g., had he vomited a substantial amount of blood), the hematocrit would have fallen, but the red blood cells and hemoglobin level would have been reduced in proportion. Because hypochromic microcytic anemia can occur in conditions other than blood loss, several tests could be ordered to confirm the original diagnosis. Which tests might be included?

4. The patient was examined by a gastroenterologist, who pointed out that black stools usually result from bleeding high in the gastrointestinal tract; if the bleeding were from lower in the gastrointestinal tract, the hemoglobin would not have been degraded to a black derivative. The physician postulated that the patient had bled from the peptic ulcer and confirmed this finding by direct visualization of the lesion through a flexible gastroscope. Although tempted to perform a transfusion, the physician instead prescribed medication to treat the ulcer, and ferrous sulfate, to be taken by mouth, to treat the anemia. What was the rationale for this maneuver?

5. How is the efficacy of therapy assessed?

CHAPTER 21

Hemostasis and Blood Coagulation

Hemophilia

A woman brings her 13-year-old son to the pediatrician's office. The boy's problems go back to the neonatal period, when he bled unduly after circumcision. When his deciduous (baby) teeth first erupted, he bit his lower lip, and the wound oozed for 2 days. As he began to crawl and walk, bruises appeared on his arms and legs. Occasionally he would sustain a nosebleed without having had an obvious injury. By the time he was 3 years of age, his parents became aware that occasionally he would have painful swelling of a joint—a knee, shoulder, wrist, or ankle—but his fingers and toes seemed spared. The joint swelling would be accompanied by exquisite tenderness; the swelling would subside in 2 to 3 days. The patient's mother states that when her son was a baby, she had noted what appeared to be blood in his stool, and the boy tells the pediatrician that twice his urine appeared red for 1 or 2 days.

Anxiously the patient's mother relates that her brother and her maternal uncle both had similar problems and were thought to be "bleeders." There is no further family history of bleeding, and there is no parental consanguinity (i.e., the patient's parents are not blood relatives). Examination of this boy reveals the presence of ecchymoses (bruises) and the inability to fully flex or extend his elbows.

A panel of four tests is ordered, with instructions to extend testing as appropriate. The four tests are a (1) platelet count, (2) prothrombin time, (3) partial thromboplastin time, and (4) bleeding time.

The patient's platelet count was found to be 260,000/µL (normal, 150,000 to 300,000/µL). This finding appears to rule out a paucity or excess of platelets as the cause of bleeding.

1. What is the role of platelets in hemostasis (the control of bleeding)?

2. What purpose is served by drawing blood into a solution of sodium citrate? What is the purpose of adding a solution of calcium chloride? Does the prothrombin time measure the intrinsic or extrinsic pathway of coagulation?

3. What mechanisms might cause the prothrombin time to be abnormally long?

4. With the given data, can you guess in general the site of the clotting abnormality in this patient?

5. Which clotting factors participate in the early steps of the intrinsic pathway of thrombin formation?

6. In reference to the patient's history, is there a discernible pattern in the way the patient's disorder might be inherited?

7. As in the case of the prothrombin time, what mechanisms might be responsible for a long partial thromboplastin time?

8. Diagnosis is made easier because deficiency of certain clotting factors either causes no symptoms or is associated only with much milder bleeding problems than the patient manifests. Which disorders can be set aside on this basis?

9. It is possible that the patient is functionally deficient in one of two clotting factors? Which are these? Can you propose a way to determine which deficiency is present?

10. Had the bleeding time been long, what diagnoses must be considered?

11. How does the bleeding time help to further delineate the diagnosis?

12. The patient's mother then added that her son's former physician had made a diagnosis of classic hemophilia. She asks, "What are the odds that his sister, now 17, is a carrier?"

THE CARDIOVASCULAR SYSTEM

Robert M. Berne
Matthew N. Levy

CHAPTER 22

The Circuitry

Hemorrhage

A 23-year-old man was in a one-car accident and was badly cut on the arms and neck. A passing motorist, who stopped to investigate the accident, pulled the victim from his overturned car and noted pulsatile bleeding from a wound in the left arm and a steady flow of blood from a wound in the neck. Before the motorist could apply pressure to the major bleeding areas, the victim had lost a lot of blood. A state trooper in a patrol car noted the accident and radioed the rescue squad, who immediately dispatched a helicopter to the site of the accident. The patient was given intravenous plasma and was flown to the nearest hospital.

1. Of the two major bleeding sites, which one was more serious and why?

2. Why was the blood flow from one bleeding site pulsatile and the other steady?

3. In the patient's vascular system, where would velocity of flow be slowest? Fastest?

4. Blood pressure fell as a result of the hemorrhage, but what was the pressure profile along the entire vascular tree (aorta to vena cavae)?

5. In which part of the circulatory system does the greatest pressure drop occur?

6. In which part of the circulatory system is most of the blood located?

CHAPTER 23

Electrical Activity of the Heart

Myocardial Infarction

A 63-year-old man suddenly felt a crushing pain beneath his sternum. He became weak and began to sweat profusely. He called his physician, who advised him to go to the hospital immediately by ambulance. The tests made at the hospital confirmed his physician's belief that the patient had suffered a "heart attack"; that is, a major coronary artery had suddenly become occluded.

1. When a coronary artery is occluded, the K^+ concentration rises in the interstitial fluid of the ischemic region (i.e., the region deprived of its blood supply) of the ventricular myocardium. What effect does the elevated K^+ concentration in the interstitial fluid have on the resting membrane potential of the myocardial cells in the ischemic zone?

2. What effect does the change in resting membrane potential have on the propagation of the cardiac impulse? Why?

3. Why might such a change in impulse propagation lead to reentrant rhythm disturbances?

This patient had cardiac rhythm disturbances within minutes after he felt the chest pain. He was given an antiarrhythmic drug that inactivated many of the fast Na^+ channels in the heart.

4. What effect would the antiarrhythmic drug have on the resting membrane potential of the myocardial cells?

5. What effect would this drug have on the upstroke of the action potential and on the propagation velocity of myocardial cells?

6. What effect does this drug have on the action potentials of the automatic cells in the sinoatrial (SA) node and on the action potential of the conduction fibers in the central (N) region of the atrioventricular (AV) node?

Soon after the patient arrived at the hospital, the activity in the vagus nerve fibers to the heart increased reflexly.

7. What electrophysiologic effects would increased vagal activity have on the automatic cells in the SA node?

8. What electrophysiologic effects would increased vagal activity have on the conduction fibers in the AV node?

About 1 hour after the coronary artery became occluded, conduction in the bundle of His ceased abruptly. The conduction block persisted for several days.

9. At approximately what rates would the atria and ventricles beat after the His bundles had been completely blocked? Where do the impulses originate that initiate the atrial and ventricular contractions in such a patient with complete AV block?

Pacing electrodes from an artificial pacemaker were inserted into the patient's right ventricle, and ventricular contractions were induced at a frequency of 75 beats/min.

10. If the artifical pacemaker suddenly ceased firing, when would the ventricles begin to contract spontaneously at their intrinsic rate? Explain.

CHAPTER 24

The Cardiac Pump

Cardiac Failure

A 70-year-old man was admitted to the hospital with shortness of breath, severe fatigue and weakness, abdominal distension, and swelling of ankles. At night he requires four pillows and often wakes up because of acute air hunger. His history revealed episodes of angina pectoris and a progressive shortness of breath with exertion for several years. On examination the chief abnormalities were slight cyanosis (bluish cast to the skin), distension of the neck veins, rapid respirations (20/min), rales (crackling sounds) at the lung bases bilaterally, an enlarged heart with slight tachycardia (110 beats/min) and a diastolic gallop rhythm (sounds like galloping horse), enlarged liver, excess fluid in the abdomen, and edema at the ankles and over the lower tibias. His blood pressure was 115/80. The chest x-ray examination showed an enlarged heart and diffuse density (indicative of fluid in the lungs) at both lung bases. An electrocardiogram (ECG) showed normal sinus rhythm, Q waves, and left axis deviation. Treatment included bed rest and administration of digitalis and a diuretic.

1. Would you expect cardiac output and stroke volume to be normal, high, or low? Why?

2. What do the distension of the neck veins and enlargement of the liver indicate? What is the mechanism?

3. Is the efficiency of the heart altered? If so, why?

4. What do you expect to find on measurement of ejection fraction and residual volume? Explain.

5. Digitalis significantly inhibits the Na/K pump. Why would this be helpful?

6. Would a calcium channel antagonist be advantageous? Why?

7. Would norepinephrine be helpful? Why?

8. Would a phlebotomy (removal of blood) or a transfusion be helpful? Why?

9. What does the diastolic gallop rhythm mean?

10. What effect does the patient's condition have on cardiac contractility? On dP/dt?

11. How important is atrial contraction for ventricular filling in this patient?

12. Is peripheral resistance changed? If so, why?

13. Why is the heart rate slightly elevated?

14. What effect would changing preload have?

15. What effect would changing afterload have?

16. Would you expect the arteriovenous oxygen difference to be normal? Why?

17. Are the force and velocity of cardiac contraction normal in this patient? How are these two variables related?

18. Is valve function normal in this patient?

19. Are the heart sounds louder, softer, or of normal intensity in this patient?

20. Why is the heart enlarged?

21. Why do the ventricles contract as a single unit?

22. How would you measure cardiac output in this patient?

23. Why is the patient short of breath?

24. Why does the patient have edema of the legs?

25. Why was a diuretic given? How does it work?

26. Should there be any dietary restrictions? If so, what?

CHAPTER 25

Regulation of the Heartbeat

Heart Block

A 48-year-old man, who engaged in regular physical exercise, went to see his physician because of recurrent headaches. Physical examination revealed that the patient had a mean heart rate of 55 beats/min. His physician noted that the patient's cardiac rhythm varied substantially with the phases of respiration; the heart rate increased during inspiration and decreased during expiration.

1. What changes in cardiac sympathetic and parasympathetic activity take place during the respiratory cycle?

2. Are the respiratory fluctuations in heart rate produced by the rhythmic changes in sympathetic activity, in parasympathetic activity, or both?

The physician diagnosed this patient's headaches as migraine. He advised the patient to take propranolol, a β-adrenergic receptor antagonist, to relieve the headaches. The physician noted that after the patient had taken the propranolol, the mean heart rate diminished very slightly, and the respiratory fluctuations in heart rate were not appreciably different from those observed before the propranolol was taken.

3. Does the failure of propranolol to induce a substantial change in mean heart rate or in the respiratory fluctuations in heart rate necessarily signify that the patient's cardiac sympathetic neural activity was negligible at the time he was being examined?

Three years later, the patient began to experience frequent episodes of chest pain on exertion. The patient's cardiologist recommended a diagnostic cardiac catheterization. His aortic pressure (Pa) and his electrocardiogram (ECG) were recorded during the procedure; one segment of the record is shown in Fig. 25-1. As the cardiac catheter was being manipulated, it initiated several premature ventricular depolarizations, one of which (designated R') is shown in this figure.

4. Why did the premature ventricular depolarization (Fig. 25-1) not affect the aortic pressure tracing?

5. Why did the ventricular contraction after the premature beat produce such a large aortic pulse pressure (difference between maximum and minimum aortic pressures)?

About 1 year later, the patient developed 2:1 atrioventricular (AV) block (i.e., only alternate cardiac impulses were propagated from atria to ventricles). The patient's ECG is shown in Fig. 25-2. Note that before the patient was given atropine (*top tracing*), those P-P intervals that include an R wave are shorter (0.7 s) than those that do not include an R wave (0.8 s). The cardiologist gave the patient test injections of propranolol and of atropine to determine the role of both divisions of the autonomic nervous system in the production of the AV block and of the alternating P-P interval durations. The cardiologist found that propranolol had little effect either on the 2:1 AV block or on the alternation of the P-P intervals. He also observed that atropine had little effect on the AV block, but it did cause the mean P-P interval to diminish (to 0.6 s), and the alternations of the P-P intervals were no longer evident (*bottom tracing*).

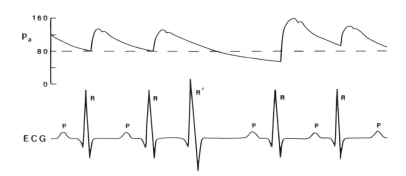

6. What is the most likely explanation for the alternating durations of the P-P intervals (Fig. 25-2)?

7. How do you explain the abolition of the alternations by atropine (Fig. 25-2), but the absence of any appreciable effect by propranolol?

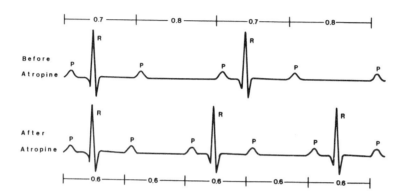

CHAPTER 26

Hemodynamics

Aortic Stenosis

A 64-year-old man, who experienced chest pain on exertion, was examined by a cardiologist. When the physician listened to the patient's chest, he heard a loud systolic murmur that was characteristic of aortic stenosis (narrowing of the aortic valve orifice). The physician advised the patient to have a cardiac catheterization, including coronary angiography.

To assess the extent of the aortic stenosis, the cardiologist first used a catheter that had an end opening. As the catheter was advanced through the aorta to a location near the aortic valve, the maximum aortic pressure during each ventricular systole was 125 mm Hg. The catheter was then removed and a different catheter inserted, which had an opening on the side of the catheter and near the tip. When the cardiologist advanced this side-hole catheter to the same position that had been reached by the preceding catheter, the maximum aortic pressure during ventricular systole was only 100 mm Hg.

1. Assuming that the patient's cardiovascular status was identical at the times that the pressure measurements were made with the end-hole and side-hole catheters, what do you estimate was the maximum velocity of blood flow through the aortic orifice?

To assess the coronary circulation in this patient, the cardiologist injected a radiopaque dye into each of the major coronary arteries. On injection of dye into the left circumflex coronary artery, fluoroscopy disclosed an arteriosclerotic lesion about 2 cm distal to the origin of that vessel. The lesion was about 1 cm in length, and the radius of the vessel lumen appeared to be reduced to about one half of normal. The mean arterial pressure (over the entire cardiac cycle) in the normal vessel proximal to the lesion was 90 mm Hg. When the catheter was advanced beyond the atherosclerotic lesion, the mean pressure was not appreciably different from that measured proximally; it was only about 1 mm Hg less than the proximal pressure.

2. Explain why the arteriosclerotic lesion, which reduced the radius of the vessel lumen by about one half, did not cause a substantial pressure drop in the artery distal to the lesion. For computational purposes, assume that (1) the resistance of the normal segments of the coronary artery is such that the pressure drop per centimeter length of vessel equals 0.1 mm Hg at the average, normal flow rate, and (2) Poiseuille's law applies to the relations between pressure and flow in both the normal and narrow segments of the artery.

3. What would be the pressure drop across the narrow segment if the radius of that segment were reduced to one fourth, rather than to one half, of normal?

The same day that the cardiologist catheterized this adult patient with aortic stenosis, a baby was also catheterized. The following hemodynamic data was obtained on the two patients:

	Adult	Baby
Mean arterial pressure (mm Hg)	95	95
Right atrial pressure (mm Hg)	5	5
Cardiac output (L/min)	5	1

4. What were the total peripheral resistances of the adult and the baby?

5. Explain the physical basis for the greater total peripheral resistance in the baby than in the adult.

CHAPTER 27

The Arterial System

Case 1: Atherosclerosis

A 43-year-old man and his father, age 80, both had heart rates of 60 beats/min, cardiac outputs of 4.8 L/min, stroke volumes of 80 ml, and total peripheral resistances of 20 mm Hg/L/min. Also, the time distributions of ventricular systole and diastole were similar in both individuals; systole occupied about 0.3 s, and diastole occupied about 0.7 s. The principal disparity in the physical characteristics of their cardiovascular systems was that the son had a very compliant arterial system, whereas the father's arterial system was very noncompliant. The son's arterial compliance (blood volume accommodated per unit change of pressure) was estimated to be about 3 ml/mm Hg, whereas that of the father was only about 0.3 ml/mm Hg.

1. What effect did the differences in arterial compliance have on the mean arterial pressures of these two individuals?

2. What effect did the differences in arterial compliance have on the systolic and diastolic arterial pressures of these two individuals?

3. What effect did the differences in arterial compliance have on the cardiac work of these two individuals?

Case 2: Heart Block

An 80-year-old man had problems with his AV conduction system, and his cardiologist decided that an artificial pacemaker was required. Immediately after the pacemaker had been installed, the cardiologist tested the effects of different pacing frequencies to determine the optimal settings for the patient. Some of the results were as follows: When the heart was paced at 60 beats/min, the patient's stroke volume was 80 ml, his cardiac output was 4.8 L/min, and his total peripheral resistance was 20 mm Hg/L/min. When the heart was paced at 100 beats/min, the stroke volume was 48 ml, his cardiac output was 4.8 L/min, and his total peripheral resistance was 20 mm Hg/L/min.

1. What was the patient's mean arterial pressure while he was being paced at heart rates of 60 and 100 beats/min?

2. What directional changes in the arterial systolic, diastolic, and pulse pressures would you expect when the paced heart rate was switched from 60 to 100 beats/min?

Case 3: Hypertension

In the course of a routine physical examination a 40-year-old man was found to have an arterial blood pressure of 175/95 mm Hg and a heart rate of 70 beats/min. The history, physical examination, and laboratory findings disclosed nothing significant other than the suggestion of slight left ventricular hypertrophy (slight increase in left ventricular mass).

1. If the patient's stroke volume, cardiac output, and central venous pressure were all normal, what hemodynamic factor must account for the subsequent development of an elevated mean arterial pressure ($\overline{P}a$)? $\overline{P}a$ is estimated to be 122 mm Hg, as determined by the equation $\overline{P}a = Pd + (Ps - Pd)/3$, where Ps and Pd are the systolic and diastolic pressures, respectively.

2. If the patient's arterial compliance is normal for his age, how do you explain that his arterial pulse pressure is abnormally large (80 mm Hg), in contrast to the average normal value of about 40 mm Hg?

CHAPTER 28

The Microcirculation and Lymphatics

Mitral Stenosis with Congestive Heart Failure

A 54-year-old woman entered the hospital with severe shortness of breath, abdominal distension, and fatigue. She has a history of rheumatic fever and has had a heart murmur since childhood. In the past 3 years she has had progressive shortness of breath and ankle edema that have required treatment with digitalis and diuretics. Despite the therapy, the patient's symptoms became much worse, and hospital admission for evaluation and treatment was recommended. Physical examination revealed a dyspneic, slightly cyanotic woman with ankle, pretibial, and sacral edema and distended neck veins. The heartbeat was completely irregular, and the heart sounds varied in intensity. Heart rate at the apex, as determined by auscultation (listening), was 100 beats/min, but as judged by the radial pulse, the heart rate was 70 beats/min. Arterial blood pressure was 100/65 mm Hg. There were loud rumbling diastolic murmurs heard best at the apex, an enlarged tender liver, ascites, and rales (crackling sounds) at both lung bases.

1. Why does the patient appear slightly cyanotic (blue)?

2. Why are neck veins distended, and is central venous pressure normal?

3. Why is the patient's blood volume increased?

4. Is velocity of peripheral blood flow increased, decreased, or normal?

5. What regulates capillary blood flow in this patient?

6. Venous pressure in the legs is elevated. Why don't the capillaries in the feet rupture?

7. What effect does the elevated intravascular pressure have on the arterioles in the feet?

8. Does the endothelium play any role in the regulation of peripheral resistance in this patient?

9. What do rales at the lung bases mean?

10. What caused the pulmonary edema in this patient?

11. Why does the patient have peripheral edema and ascites?

12. Is there impairment of water and/or sodium movement between the vascular and the extravascular compartments?

13. Is O_2 and CO_2 exchange between blood and tissue normal?

14. Are oncotic forces in the patient's blood normal?

15. If all capillaries are open, would this affect the formation of edema?

16. How would large molecules move between blood and tissue?

17. What role do the lymphatics play in this patient?

18. Why were the heart sounds irregular?

19. Why were the heart sounds of varying intensity, and why was the heart rate at the apex by auscultation different from that at the wrist by palpation?

CHAPTER 29

The Peripheral Circulation and Its Control

Thromboangiitis Obliterans

A 50-year-old man went to see his physician because of pain in the calf muscles of both legs when he walked moderate distances, especially uphill; the pain would subside when he rested. The pain had been insidious in onset and had recently occurred more frequently, even after shorter walks. The patient had smoked three packs of cigarettes a day for the past 34 years. Physical examination was essentially normal except for the absence of dorsalis pedis and posterior tibial pulses in both feet. X-ray examinations revealed arterial calcification of lower leg arteries and significant obstruction of the arteries above the knees.

1. Is the main resistance to blood flow in the patient's legs the same as in a healthy person?

2. Is the vascular smooth muscle functioning normally in this patient?

3. How would the arterioles of this patient respond to stimulation of sympathetic nerve fibers to the legs?

4. Which ion is of greatest importance in contraction of the vascular smooth muscle?

5. What is autoregulation of blood flow, and does it operate in this patient's legs?

6. In which vascular beds is the myogenic mechanism for blood flow regulation most important in healthy individuals? In this patient?

7. How may the endothelium be involved in the local regulation of blood flow in healthy people? In this patient?

8. Why does he experience calf muscle pain in response to moderate walking?

9. What is metabolic regulation of blood flow, and how does it apply in this patient?

10. How are his basal tone, active hyperemia, and reactive hyperemia affected?

11. What is the role of the sympathetic nerves in regulating leg blood flow?

12. How do resistance and capacitance vessels differ with respect to sensitivity to sympathetic nerve stimulation and to metabolic vasoactive mediators in the healthy person and in this patient?

13. Would sympathetic denervation be helpful in this patient?

14. What effect would a peripheral vasodilator, such as acetylcholine or adenosine, have on this patient?

15. What effect would a peripheral constrictor, such as norepinephrine have?

16. What is responsible for the short-term and long-term maintenance of blood pressure?

17. What would happen to the patient's respiration, blood pressure, and leg blood flow if he breathed a mixture of 10% CO_2, 21% O_2, and 69% N_2?

18. What would happen to his respiration, blood pressure, and leg blood flow if he breathed a mixture of 10% O_2 and 90% N_2?

19. Muscle blood vessels are under dual control (neural and local metabolic). Which of these factors predominates at rest and during exercise in the arms and legs of this patient?

CHAPTER 30

Control of Cardiac Output: Coupling of Heart and Blood Vessels

Acute Myocardial Infarction

A 68-year-old woman was admitted to the coronary intensive care unit with the diagnosis of acute myocardial infarction. Soon after admission, she was resting comfortably, and seemed to be doing well, except for occasional premature ventricular contractions. Her arterial blood pressure, central venous pressure, and other vital signs were normal, except that her heart rate was moderately increased. On the second hospital day, the cardiac monitor showed that the patient suddenly developed ventricular fibrillation, her arterial blood pressure dropped precipitously to about 8 mm Hg, and her central venous pressure, which had been about 3 mm Hg, rapidly rose to about 8 mm Hg.

1. Why did the development of ventricular fibrillation lead to a rise in the patient's central venous pressure?

2. Why was the fall in arterial blood pressure so much greater than the rise in central venous pressure?

This patient was successfully resuscitated, and her condition improved rapidly. She was discharged from the hospital 10 days after admission. However, 4 months later she noticed that she frequently became short of breath on mild exertion. Her physician made the diagnosis of congestive heart failure and recommended that she be treated with a new, experimental drug that improved myocardial contractility. The patient's cardiac output before treatment was 4.3 L/min, and her central venous pressure was 12 mm Hg. One hour after she had received the new drug, her cardiac output had increased to 5.2 L/min, and her central venous pressure had diminished to 6 mm Hg.

3. Explain how a drug that acts specifically to enhance myocardial contractility can increase cardiac output and decrease central venous pressure.

4. Is an increase in cardiac output in the presence of a reduction in the ventricular filling pressure (central venous pressure) incompatible with the Frank-Starling mechanism?

The experimental drug given to improve myocardial contractility did not prove to be sufficiently efficacious. Therefore her physician decided to use a more conventional treatment, namely an *afterload reducing agent*. This type of drug acts mainly to relax arteriolar smooth muscle cells. This treatment effectively relieved her shortness of breath on exertion. However, she frequently noticed that on arising from the recumbent position, she felt very light-headed and sometimes had difficulty remaining upright. Her physician found that the patient's arterial blood pressure was normal while she was recumbent, but that when she stood up, her blood pressure decreased substantially; this phenomenon is called *orthostatic hypotension*.

5. In healthy individuals receiving no drug therapy, what changes in cardiac output and arterial blood pressure occur when they assume the upright posture?

6. What compensatory mechanisms are called into play normally?

7. What effect does the vascular smooth muscle relaxant drug have on these overall hemodynamic reactions in the patient who developed orthostatic hypotension when she assumed the upright posture?

Two years later, this patient developed serious problems with her AV conduction system, and she had an artificial pacemaker installed. When her heart was paced at a rate of 60 beats/min, her stroke volume was 80 ml; but when her heart was paced at 100 beats/min, her stroke volume was only 48 ml.

8. What was the cardiac output when the heart was paced artificially at each frequency?

9. How do stroke volume and cardiac output vary as a function of the frequency of cardiac contraction (heart rate)?

CHAPTER 31

Special Circulations

Coronary Artery Disease and Bypass Surgery—Familial Dysbetalipoproteinemia

A 42-year-old man entered the hospital because of multiple complaints. His family history reveals that his father and his two older brothers died of coronary artery disease in their midforties. For several years the patient has had increasing bouts of angina pectoris (which was relieved by nitroglycerin), pain in the calves of his legs when he climbs stairs, and two episodes of transient cerebral ischemia within the past month. Physical examination was not remarkable, except for xanthoma (yellow-orange fatty deposits) on his palms and around his knees and elbows and absence of pulses in the feet. Angiograms showed extensive atheromatous disease in the abdominal aorta and in the carotid, coronary, mesenteric, femoral, and popliteal arteries with almost complete blockage of blood flow in two coronary arteries. Because of his leg problems, he was given a cardiac stress test with an intravenous infusion of adenosine, instead of exercise on a treadmill. The test elicited angina and ST segment changes indicative of myocardial ischemia. Blood cholesterol level and triglycerides were elevated, and genetic analysis revealed that he had familial dysbetalipoproteinemia.

After a thoracotomy for coronary bypass surgery, he was heparinized, placed on a pump-oxygenator, and had potassium chloride injected into his coronary arteries and ice-cold saline applied to his heart. After completion of the coronary bypass surgery, he was hypotensive when taken off the pump-oxygenator and was treated with a vasoconstrictor to maintain a normal blood pressure. Were it not for the extensive atherosclerosis in his femoral arteries and abdominal aorta, he would have had a counterpulsation device placed in his abdominal aorta via a femoral artery. This device consists of a long inflatable balloon. Inflation and deflation are synchronized with the heartbeat; the balloon is inflated during diastole and deflated during systole.

A week after the bypass surgery, his coronary blood flow, as measured by the thermodilution technique, was found to be improved.

1. What is the rationale of the adenosine stress test?

2. Why was potassium chloride injected, and why was ice-cold saline applied to the heart when the patient was placed on the pump-oxygenator?

3. Why would a counterpulsation device have been beneficial during the postoperative recovery period?

4. How is thermodilution used to measure coronary blood flow?

5. What are the physical factors that affect coronary blood flow in this patient?

6. What role do the sympathetic nerves play in the regulation of his coronary blood flow?

7. What are the chemical factors that influence his coronary blood flow?

8. Would epicardial and endocardial blood flow be affected equally?

9. How does nitroglycerin relieve the patient's angina pectoris? What effect does this drug have on blood pressure and skin blood flow?

10. What causes the development of collateral vessels in this patient's heart?

11. With central activation of the sympathetic nervous system, how do vascular beds in heart, skeletal muscle, skin, gastrointestinal tract, kidney, and brain differ?

12. What effect would elevation of environmental temperature have on this patient?

13. What effect would exposure to cold have on this patient?

14. What role do the venous valves play in the different vascular beds of this patient?

15. The patient experienced pain in the right leg when climbing stairs. What effect might this have on regional cerebral blood flow?

16. What happens to gastrointestinal and liver blood flow and digestive activity when the patient exercises (runs)?

17. What effect would CO_2 inhalation have on his cerebral blood flow?

18. What effect would hypoxia have on his cerebral blood flow?

19. What effect does the patient's atherosclerosis have on cerebral blood flow and arteriolar resistance?

20. If this patient had a patent ductus arteriosus, what kind of murmur would he have and why?

CHAPTER 32

Interplay of Central and Peripheral Factors in the Control of the Circulation

Case 1: Exercise Tolerance Evaluation

A well-trained, 20-year-old track star is in excellent health and has often run a mile in under 4 minutes. As part of a large group study of young athletes engaged in endurance sports, he enters the exercise laboratory for evaluation of his physical condition during treadmill exercise.

1. What are the key cardiovascular changes that occur at the starting block during an actual race?

2. As the treadmill is speeded up, what happens to heart rate, peripheral resistance, skin blood flow, cardiac output, and blood flow distribution?

3. Is an increase in $PaCO_2$ responsible for the increase in respiration, heart rate, and cardiac output?

4. Why does blood flow to the leg muscles increase?

5. Is there a change in leg muscle interstitial pressure during the exercise?

6. What happens to arterial and central venous oxygen levels?

7. What influences venous return during the exercise?

8. What happens to stroke volume and blood pressure?

9. What factors affect skin blood flow and body temperatures during the exercise?

10. What limits the runner's performance, and how does training improve it?

Case 2: Hemorrhage and Shock

Two soldiers received similar wounds during a battle, and they each lost a substantial amount of blood. Neither was able to receive any treatment other than medication for pain. Each soldier was noted to have a mean arterial blood pressure of about 50 mm Hg shortly after being wounded. Their blood pressures gradually increased for the first 2 hours. Thereafter, soldier A's blood pressure continued to improve, and within 4 or 5 hours, his blood pressure was almost normal. He ultimately survived. However, soldier B's blood pressure reached a peak value of only about 65 mm Hg a few hours after he had been wounded. His blood pressure then gradually declined, and he died about 10 hours after being wounded.

1. Cite the various compensatory mechanisms that may have contributed to the recovery of soldier A.

2. Cite the various decompensatory mechanisms that may have contributed to the demise of soldier B.

3. Assume that a specific, potent positive inotropic drug was available; that is, the drug could improve myocardial contractility substantially, but it would have no appreciable effects on the vasculature. Discuss the potential efficacy of such a drug if it were given to either soldier during the first hour after the injury.

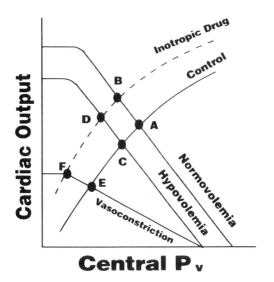

THE RESPIRATORY SYSTEM

Lawrence Martin

CHAPTER 33

Structure and Function of the Respiratory System

Obstructive Airway Disease

A 50-year-old man comes to the pulmonary laboratory for evaluation of chronic shortness of breath. He has smoked one pack of cigarettes a day for 30 years. His arterial blood is analyzed for pH, partial pressure of oxygen (PaO_2), partial pressure of carbon dioxide ($PaCO_2$), percentage saturation of hemoglobin with oxygen (SaO_2), and hemoglobin content; the results are shown below. The patient is at sea level and breathing ambient air (21% oxygen). His respiratory rate is 25 respirations per minute, and tidal volume is 400 ml.

pH	7.47
PaO_2	60 mm Hg
SaO_2	90%
$PaCO_2$	30 mm Hg
Hemoglobin	14 g/dl blood

1. What do PaO_2 and SAO_2 signify, and how are they related?

2. What is the total oxygen content in the patient's arterial blood? Do you need to use a hemoglobin-oxygen equilibrium curve to answer this question?

3. Is there sufficient information to calculate minute ventilation, dead space ventilation, and alveolar ventilation? If so, make the calculation; if not, state why not. Can you discern from the respiratory rate and/or tidal volume if he is hyperventilating?

4. From the alveolar ventilation equation below, state what determines the alveolar PCO_2 and under what circumstances it might change.

$$PaCO_2 = \frac{VCO_2 \times 0.863}{VA}$$

5. Is this patient's alveolar ventilation, relative to CO_2 production, more or less than normal? How is the answer to this question used to determine if a patient is hyperventilating or hypoventilating? What is the clinical significance of this information?

6. What is his calculated PAO_2? (Use the alvolar gas equation below. As is customary, assume that PCO_2 measured in arterial blood [$PaCO_2$] equals mean alveolar PCO_2 [$PACO_2$]. Also, assume his respiratory quotient is 0.8.)

$$PAO_2 = PIO_2 - PaCO_2 \left[FIO_2 + \frac{(1 - FIO_2)}{R}\right]$$

Where $PIO_2 = FIO_2$ (barometric pressure - 47 mm Hg)

7. Subtract PaO_2 from the calculated PAO_2. Is the value for $(PAO_2 - PaO_2)$ abnormally increased? What is the significance of an increased $(PAO_2 - PaO_2)$?

8. What is your overall interpretation of the blood gas data, in terms of the patient's oxygenation and ventilation?

The patient next undergoes tests of mechanical lung function. The following lung volumes and capacities are measured. (Percentages of predicted values are shown; any lung volume or capacity between 80% to 120% of predicted is considered in the normal range.)

Forced vital capacity (FVC) = 3 L = 75% of predicted
Forced expiratory volume in one second (FEV-1) = 1.6 L = 55% of predicted
Total lung capacity = 7.8 L = 130% of predicted
Residual volume = 2.8 L = 140% of predicted

9. What is the difference between a lung volume and a lung capacity?

10. How do you interpret the lung volume and capacity information? What do you think is the nature of his clinical problem?

11. Which of the lung volume and lung capacity measurements cannot be determined by spirometry alone, but requires an additional technique (such as inert gas dilution)?

CHAPTER 34

Mechanical Properties in Breathing

Pulmonary Edema

A 50-year-old woman is in intensive care for treatment of pulmonary edema caused by heart failure. Edema fluid is in both the interstitial and alveolar spaces of her lungs. For the moment she is breathing on her own, (i.e., she is not connected to a mechanical ventilator). Her respiratory rate is 30 per minute. Previously, she had normal lungs.

1. Based on this limited information, how would you characterize the following parameters as high, low, or normal? State your reasons.

   Total lung capacity
   Surface tension
   Lung compliance
   Work of breathing
   Airway resistance

After a few hours her condition deteriorates, and she is mechanically ventilated. The ventilator delivers 12 breaths/min, and tidal volume is 500 ml. The ventilator measures airway pressure at the end of each delivered tidal volume, at a point of "no air flow"; at this point, airway pressure is 30 cm H_2O. The ventilator then allows her to passively exhale, and airway pressure returns to zero (atmospheric).

2. What is her thoracic compliance (state the units)? Is this a measurement of lung, chest wall, or lung plus chest wall compliance? In measuring thoracic compliance, what is the importance of obtaining the peak pressure at a point of no air flow?

3. A separate set of measurements is taken during air flow. During inhalation she has an airway opening pressure (PaO) of 35 cm H_2O, an alveolar pressure (PA) of 25 cm H_2O, and an air flow of 1 L/sec. What is the calculated airway resistance? Is this a normal value? Do you think this measurement reflects her true airway resistance?

The patient recovers completely. Two months later she returns to the pulmonary function laboratory. She is asked to inhale fully, then exhale as forcefully and fully as possible, and then resume normal breathing. During the test, the volume of air exhaled and the rate of air flow are measured.

4. What is the term for the volume of air that is (a) in her lungs at the point of maximal inhalation; (b) exhaled from full inhalation to full exhalation; and (c) in her lungs at the point of full exhalation?

5. At what point in this maneuver is her air flow the fastest? If she did not inhale maximally before commencing this maneuver, would her maximal air flow be the same, higher, or lower than maximal inhalation? Explain your answer.

6. What is the term for the volume of air in her lungs at the end of quiet, normal breathing? How does it compare with a typical normal value? What is her intrapleural pressure at this point, relative to atmospheric pressure (negative or positive)? Explain the elastic recoil forces acting at this point. If one side of her chest wall is punctured, what will happen to the lung on that side, and why?

7. Patients with recurrent episodes of pulmonary edema sometimes don't recover fully, but may develop pulmonary fibrosis, or chronic lung scarring. Fibrotic lungs differ from emphysematous lungs. How do each of the following parameters compare to normal (increased, decreased, or no change)?

	Emphysema	Pulmonary fibrosis
Elastic recoil		
Compliance		
Total lung capacity		
Functional residual capacity		
Forced vital capacity		
Residual volume		
Minute ventilation		
Oxygen tension in arterial blood		
Carbon dioxide tension in arterial blood		

CHAPTER 35

Pulmonary and Bronchial Circulations: Ventilation/Perfusion Ratios

Case 1: Pneumonia with Severe Hypoxia

Mr. D., a previously healthy 35-year-old man, is seen in the emergency department for cough and shortness of breath; the evaluation takes place at sea level. Chest x-ray examination shows a large infiltrate, consistent with the clinical diagnosis of pneumonia, in his left lung. When the patient is breathing ambient air (FIO_2 is 0.21), his arterial PO_2 (PaO_2) is 52 mm Hg, $PaCO_2$ is 39 mm Hg, and pH is 7.42. Minute ventilation is 12 L/min.

1. Listed below are the major physiologic mechanisms that can diminish PaO_2. For each mechanism, explain how it may or may not play a role in causing *this* patient's low PaO_2.

    Ventilation/perfusion imbalance
    Right to left intrapulmonary shunt
    Diffusion barrier to gas transfer
    Hypoventilation

2. Does this minute ventilation, together with the $PaCO_2$, indicate an increase in wasted ventilation? How is an increase in wasted ventilation explained by ventilation/perfusion imbalance?

3. While he is breathing 50% oxygen via a face mask, the following blood gas results are obtained: PaO_2 is 65 mm Hg, $PaCO_2$ is 35 mm Hg, and pH is 7.46. Do these results change your assessment of the physiologic cause of his hypoxemia?

Mr. D. is admitted to intensive care and continues to manifest severe hypoxemia. Overnight the pneumonia spreads to involve his entire left lung, but it spares the right lung. He is now receiving 100% inspired oxygen via face mask, plus broad spectrum antibiotics. He remains awake and alert, and breathes at a rate of 28 times per minute. Arterial blood gases show the following: PaO_2 is 60 mm Hg, and $PaCO_2$ is 30 mm Hg.

4. Based on the above information, what is the approximate percentage of the right to left shunt?

5. These blood gases are obtained while he is lying on his left side. His physician, concerned about the low PO_2, is considering tracheal intubation and mechanical ventilation. However, the physician first decides to change the patient's body position to improve PaO_2. What is the change asked for, and why?

Mr. D. appears in the emergency department a year later. He took an overdose of sleeping pills and is comatose. His chest x-ray examination is clear and shows no residual of the pneumonia. Vital signs reveal a normal blood pressure, pulse is 100 beats/min and regular, and respirations are 6 per minute and shallow. A friend states that the patient has been despondent over domestic problems, and he has no prior history of drug overdose. Arterial blood gases show that pH is 7.34, PaO_2 is 55 mm Hg, and $PaCO_2$ is 70 mm Hg.

6. With reference to the same four mechanisms of hypoxemia listed in question 1, explain the patient's low PaO_2.

7. What is the principal physiologic process that needs correction in this patient: ventilation or oxygenation? What would be appropriate treatment?

Case 2: Lung Cancer

A 60-year-old man undergoes surgery to remove his entire right lung as treatment for lung cancer. His left lung is normal. Assume that, after full recovery, he maintains the same cardiac output and alveolar ventilation as before, and the same CO_2 production. What is the expected change, if any, in each of the following parameters?

1. Pulmonary artery pressure

2. Pulmonary vascular resistance

3. PaO_2

4. $PaCO_2$

5. V/Q balance

6. Exercise tolerance

CHAPTER 36

Transport of Oxygen and Carbon Dioxide: Tissue Oxygenation

Case 1: Carbon Monoxide Poisoning

A young man is rescued from a fire and brought to the emergency department (located at sea level). The patient is unconscious, but his vital signs (heart rate, blood pressure, respiratory rate) are stable. Below are arterial blood gas data, from a sample drawn while he is breathing 100% oxygen.

$Pa_{O_2} = 190$ mm Hg $Pa_{CO_2} = 36$ mm Hg   COHb = 40%
pH = 7.47 $Sa_{O_2} = 60\%$

1. What is the relative position of his HbO_2 equilibrium curve compared to normal? Is the curve pushed upward or downward? Is it shifted to the left or right? Explain the effect of the changes in his HbO_2 equilibrium curve on:

   - The amount of oxygen delivered *from* the lungs *to* the tissue capillaries
   - The amount of oxygen delivered *from* the tissue capillaries *to* the individual tissue cells

2. Is his Pa_{O_2} less than, equal to, or higher than expected under the circumstances (100% inspired oxygen, normal Pa_{CO_2})? Explain your answer.

3. What is the relative affinity of CO and O_2 for hemoglobin? Based on this information, how should a victim of CO poisoning be treated?

4. Describe and explain how each of the following conditions would affect this patient's Pa_{O_2}, Sa_{O_2}, and arterial oxygen content. Assume that each condition occurs alone (i.e., nothing else is abnormal).

Condition	Pa_{O_2}	Sa_{O_2}	O_2 content
Anemia			
Excess CO			
Fever			
Acidosis			
Alkalosis			
Hypoventilation			
Hyperventilation			
V/Q imbalance			
High altitude			

Case 2: Emphysema with Respiratory Failure

A 60-year-old woman is in the intensive care unit for treatment of respiratory tract failure. Her underlying disease is emphysema, caused by years of smoking. Her trachea is intubated, and the tube is connected to a mechanical ventilator that has taken over her breathing. The fraction of inspired oxygen is 0.6. The machine-delivered tidal volume is 700 ml and the rate is 12 breaths/minute. She is afebrile and has normal blood pressure. The following data are obtained:

From arterial blood:

pH = 7.5 PCO_2 = 35 mm Hg
PaO_2 = 60 mm Hg SaO_2 = 92%
FIO_2 = 0.6   Hemoglobin = 9 g/dl

From a cardiac catheter in the pulmonary artery:

Cardiac output = 5 L/min
PvO_2 = 40 mm Hg (mixed venous PO_2)
SvO_2 = 73% (mixed venous oxygen saturation)

1. Write the formula you would use to calculate the following:

    a. Arterial oxygen content
    b. Arterial oxygen delivery
    c. Venous oxygen content
    d. Oxygen uptake
    e. Venous oxygen delivery

2. Assuming that all other factors remain the same, explain the result of each of the following changes on her *arterial oxygen content* and *arterial oxygen delivery*. In each instance where the HbO_2 equilibrium curve is altered, state whether the P_{50} is lower or higher than normal.

    a. Increase in $PaCO_2$ to 50 mm Hg
    b. Increase in body temperature to 101° F
    c. Increase in pH to 7.58
    d. Increase in PaO_2 to 80 mm Hg
    e. Increase in hemoglobin to 12 g/dl blood
    f. Decrease in cardiac output to 4 L/min

3. Based on the information provided:

    a. Approximately what percentage of oxygen delivered to the systemic tissue capillaries is taken up and metabolized by the tissues?

    b. Approximately what percentage of oxygen delivered to the systemic tissue capillaries returns to the right heart?

CHAPTER 37

Control of Breathing

Case 1: Hyperventilation and Sleep Apnea

Mrs. S. is a 40-year-old woman who has been obese since her early 20s. She now weighs 290 pounds and is 5 feet, 2 inches tall. For the past 6 months she has become increasingly short of breath with any exertion. On examination she appears to be a pleasant, alert woman in no apparent distress, and she breathes 24 times a minute. In addition to shortness of breath, which she feels just walking across the room, she complains of falling asleep very easily during the day. In fact she no longer drives because a month earlier she fell asleep at the wheel but was uninjured. Her chest x-ray examination and electrocardiogram show no abnormalities. In the pulmonary function laboratory, she has the following blood gas and spirometry values (all at sea level).

Arterial blood gas and hemoglobin (while she breathed room air)

pH = 7.35
$Paco_2$ = 67 mm Hg
Pao_2 = 58 mm Hg
Sao_2 = 86%
Hemoglobin content = 15 g/dl

Spirometry data

FVC = 78% of predicted
FEV-1 = 78% of predicted
FEV-1/FVC = 100%

1. How do you interpret these blood gas values? Is she hypoventilating? Why is her Pao_2 low?

2. How do you interpret the spirometry values? Does she have restrictive or obstructive mechanical impairment? Would you assess the impairment to be mild, moderate, or severe?

3. Do you believe the degree of mechanical impairment is sufficient to explain the elevated $Paco_2$? If not, what is the most likely explanation?

Mrs. S. is admitted to the hospital for further evaluation and for a trial of oxygen therapy. While she receives 2 L/min of oxygen through a nasal tube, her blood analyses show the following:

pH = 7.33
$Paco_2$ = 71 mm Hg
Pao_2 = 88 mm Hg
Sao_2 = 92%

The first night in the hospital she undergoes a sleep study. She is connected to machines that continually monitor her chest wall movements, oxygen saturation, air flow through mouth and nostrils, and electro-encephalogram (EEG). Because her oxygen saturation is low while she breathes room air, she receives oxygen, at a flow rate of 2 L/min while she sleeps. Frequently while she sleeps, the following abnormal pattern is observed: air flow ceases while her chest wall movements increase. This abnormal pattern recurs throughout the night; each time it lasts between 10 and 45 seconds; each occasion ends with Mrs. S. making a loud snort or snoring sound, at which point air flow resumes. During these periods of absent air flow, her oxygen saturation falls, often to as low as 72%.

4. What type of sleep problem does this pattern indicate? What is the cause? What type of treatment would overcome this problem?

Two years later, Mrs. S. is admitted to the intensive care unit. She now weighs 320 pounds and has not seen a physician for at least a year. On examination she is lethargic and barely arousable. She has edema in both legs. Her hemoglobin content is increased to 19 g/dl (polycythemia). Arterial blood analyses while the patient breathes room air show the following:

pH = 7.29
Pa_{CO_2} = 70 mm Hg
Pa_{O_2} = 38 mm Hg
Sa_{O_2} = 74%

5. What is her current problem and its cause? Why is her hemoglobin content increased? What should the treatment be at this point?

She improves after 2 weeks of intensive care and leaves the hospital 30 pounds lighter. Her home-going regimen consists of oxygen at 2 L/min through an intranasal tube, plus a device (a continuous positive airway pressure mask) that forces air through her nostrils under pressure while she sleeps. A strict diet is also prescribed. A month after leaving the hospital, she returns to the laboratory for further evaluation. She now weighs 280 pounds. Arterial blood gases, pH, and hemoglobin are rechecked while she does not receive supplemental oxygen.

Arterial pH/blood gas and hemoglobin (while breathing room air)

pH = 7.37
Pa_{CO_2} = 60 mm Hg
Pa_{O_2} = 61 mm Hg
Sa_{O_2} = 89%
Hemoglobin content = 15.5 g/dl

6. A CO_2 response graph is plotted by having her breathe a low concentration of CO_2 and measuring her minute ventilation against the exhaled, end-tidal P_{CO_2} (which represents the arterial blood P_{CO_2}). During this test she is also given supplemental oxygen so that her Pa_{O_2} stays in a normal range. From her history, what type of CO_2 response curve do you expect to see?

Case 2: Effects of High Altitude

You and some friends decide to journey to the top of a mountain that is 16,000 feet above sea level. Assume that you reside, and start your trip, at sea level, and that it takes 2 days to reach the summit. Describe how each of the following parameters will change during your journey, and explain each change.

1. FIO_2
2. Barometric pressure
3. Pa_{O_2}
4. Pa_{CO_2}
5. P_{50}
6. Pulmonary artery pressure

Near the summit, at 14,000 feet, you meet villagers who have lived at this altitude all their lives. Compare the following parameters in the mountain dwellers to people who live near sea level:

7. Hemoglobin content
8. Hypoxic ventilatory response
9. Hypercapnic ventilatory response

At the summit, one member of the climbing party becomes very short of breath and complains of severe headache.

10. Assume you have only a basic first aid kit, which does not contain any supply of oxygen. What is the treatment of choice?

THE GASTROINTESTINAL SYSTEM

Howard C. Kutchai

CHAPTER 38

Gastrointestinal Motility

Achalasia

A 42-year-old woman is admitted to the hospital because of difficulty in swallowing solid foods; liquids are less difficult to swallow. Chest pain follows eating, and the patient frequently regurgitates swallowed food after a meal. When the recumbent patient is observed by fluoroscopy after a barium swallow, her lower esophagus is seen to be somewhat dilated, but her upper esophagus is of normal caliber. Subsequent swallows initiated by the patient do not cause the barium to be cleared from the esophagus as rapidly as in a normal individual. Rather, it appears that the lower esophageal sphincter (LES) relaxes very transiently, allowing small amounts of barium to empty into the stomach. Administration of amyl nitrate accelerates clearance of barium from the esophagus. The transient openings of the LES do not bear any simple temporal relationship to the swallows initiated by the patient. Esophageal manometric studies of the patient are then undertaken. The coordinated peristaltic wave that is observed in the esophagus of a normal individual after a swallow does not occur in this patient. Rather, each swallow elicits a low pressure increase in the esophagus; the pressure increase occurs almost simultaneously at various places along the length of the esophagus. The resting pressure in the LES is about 60 mm Hg, and the LES pressure decreases to about 45 mm Hg after a swallow. The patient is treated by dilating the LES by brief, forceful inflations of a pneumatic device. After this procedure, the patient's ability to swallow solid food is dramatically improved. Fifteen months after the dilation, the patient returns with the complaint that swallowing has again become difficult.

1. What appears abnormal on fluoroscopic examination after a barium swallow?

2. What esophageal malfunctions might account for these observations?

3. What is learned from the patient's response to amyl nitrate administration?

4. What abnormalities are revealed by manometric studies?

5. What physiologic malfunctions are suggested by the manometric studies?

6. Why does the increase in pressure after a swallow occur at the same time at different locations along the esophagus?

7. Why did the forceful dilation of the LES enhance the ability of the patient to swallow solid food?

8. Why did the patient's symptoms recur?

9. What therapeutic options remain when the patient's symptoms reappear?

CHAPTER 39

Gastrointestinal Secretions

Hyperacidity with Duodenal Ulcer and Gastrinoma

A 25-year-old woman enters the hospital with persistent diarrhea and abdominal pain. An upper gastrointestinal radiologic series suggests the presence of a duodenal ulcer, which is confirmed by endoscopy. The patient's basal rate of secretion of gastric HCl is about 12 mmole/hr (the normal range is 1 to 5 mmole/hr). The patient's serum gastrin is 1145 pg/ml (the normal range is 50 to 150 pg/ml). When the patient's gastric juice is removed via a nasogastric tube during a 24-hour period, the diarrhea is corrected. The patient also has moderate steatorrhea (excess fat in the stool). A sample of the mucosa of the patient's gastric fundus is taken via the endoscope. Histologic examination of the mucosal specimen reveals that the gastric glands are more numerous than normal and have a higher density of parietal cells than normal. After a test meal, the patient's serum gastrin level does not increase significantly. In the average normal individual the same meal produces a doubling of serum gastrin. Intravenous infusion of secretin results in a peak serum gastrin level that is three times the basal level. In normal individuals, infusion of secretin has little effect on serum gastrin; the most common response is a slight decrease in serum gastrin. The patient's rate of HCl secretion can be brought to below normal levels by treatment with the H_2 receptor blocker cimetidine. However, the dose of cimetidine required to do this is several times greater than that usually used for patients with duodenal ulcer, and the drug must be administered four to six times daily to suppress HCl secretion effectively. Administration of a cholinergic antagonist enhances the therapeutic effect of the cimetidine. A single daily dose of the H^+, K^+-ATPase blocker omeprazole is effective in bringing HCl secretion to below normal rates.

1. Why might the patient have an elevated basal rate of gastric HCl secretion?

2. How would you expect the patient's rate of pepsinogen secretion to compare with normal?

3. Why does the patient have a duodenal ulcer?

4. Why doesn't the patient have a gastric ulcer?

5. What abnormalities might lead to elevated serum gastrin levels?

6. Why does the patient have steatorrhea?

7. What causes the patient to have diarrhea?

8. Why does the patient have an increased density of parietal cells in her fundic mucosa?

9. Why does the patient not have a significant increase in serum gastrin after a test meal?

10. Why does the patient have such a large increase in serum gastrin after intravenous infusion of secretin?

11. Why is cimetidine effective? Why are such large and frequent doses of cimetidine required?

12. How might a cholinergic antagonist enhance the effectiveness of cimetidine in reducing HCl secretion by the patient's gastric mucosa?

13. How does omeprazole decrease the patient's rate of HCl secretion? Why is only one dose per day required?

14. What options exist for the long-term management of this patient's care?

CHAPTER 40

Digestion and Absorption

Tryptophan Transport Dysfunction—Hartnup's Syndrome

A 12-year-old boy is referred to a dermatologist because of a skin rash reminiscent of pellagra. The rash appears occasionally and is exacerbated by exposure to the sun. The rash is confined to the face, back of the neck, backs of the hands and wrists, external surfaces of arms and legs, anterior surfaces of knees, and dorsal surfaces of the feet. The patient's diet contains sufficient niacin and calories, but is low in protein. The patient is not frankly malnourished. The parents of the patient have not reported similar skin rashes, but a sister of the patient has suffered from similar photosensitive skin rashes. The urine of the patient contains most of the neutral amino acids in levels from 5 to 20 times their levels in the urine of normal individuals. These amino acids include alanine, asparagine, glutamine, histidine, isoleucine, leucine, phenylalanine, serine, threonine, tyrosine, and valine. The patient's urine does not contain elevated levels of basic or acidic amino acids, nor elevated levels of the neutral amino acids glycine, methionine, or cystine. The patient's plasma levels of individual amino acids are not abnormal. When the patient is fed partially hydrolyzed casein (polypeptides), the plasma levels of the neutral amino acids rise in the plasma several hours later, as is the case for normal individuals. However, when the patient is fed a mixture of amino acids, there is only a very small rise in the plasma levels of those neutral amino acids that are elevated in the patient's urine. The patient is treated daily with oral doses of niacin (200 mg/kg) and the episodic skin rash disappears. With this regimen, the patient is asymptomatic.

1. What might account for the higher concentrations of neutral amino acids found in the patient's urine?

2. What might account for the failure of the plasma levels of these same amino acids to rise after feeding the patient a mixture of all the amino acids?

3. Why do the plasma levels of these neutral amino acids rise after the patient is fed partially hydrolyzed casein?

4. Why does the patient apparently have a deficit of niacin, despite having an amount of niacin in his diet that would be sufficient for a normal individual?

5. What bearing might the patient's low-protein diet have on his condition?

6. Why is the patient not malnourished?

7. Because the symptoms of this disorder resemble pellagra, and the symptoms are alleviated by feeding the patient elevated doses of niacin, why is the patient's problem not simply called pellagra?

SECTION
VIII

THE KIDNEY

Bruce A. Stanton
Bruce M. Koeppen

CHAPTER 41

Elements of Renal Function

Case 1: Poststreptococcal Glomerulonephritis

A 17-year-old girl develops poststreptococcal glomerulonephritis. In this condition the glomeruli are damaged by an acute inflammatory reaction. This inflammatory response damages the filtration barrier, and the integrity of the capillary endothelium and the net negative charge on the glomerular basement membrane are lost.

Which of the following substances would appear in greater quantity in the urine of this girl?

A. Red blood cells
B. Glucose
C. Sodium
D. Proteins

Case 2: Filtration, Secretion, and Reabsorption

A healthy volunteer participates in a clinical research project designed to examine the renal handling of various substances. The results of the project are given below. Fill in the chart and determine how substances A, B, C, and D are handled by the kidneys (i.e., filtered only, filtered and reabsorbed, or filtered and secreted). It is known that 50% of substance B is bound to plasma protein, and 75% of substance D is bound to plasma protein. Neither substance A nor C is protein bound. The urine flow rate is 0.5 ml/min.

Substance	Urine [x] (mg/ml)	Plasma [x]* (mg/ml)	$U_x \times \dot{V}$ (mg/min)	Clearance (ml/min)	Filtered load (mg/min)	Transport rate (mg/min)
Inulin	5.5	0.025	_____	_____	_____	_____
A	0.8	0.040	_____	_____	_____	_____
B	7.5	0.068	_____	_____	_____	_____
C	11.0	0.010	_____	_____	_____	_____
D	10.0	0.060	_____	_____	_____	_____

*Plasma [x] represents the total concentration (i.e., bound plus unbound).

Case 3: Micturition

A 21-year-old man is in an automobile accident. His spinal cord is injured, resulting in paralysis of his legs and loss of sensation from the waist down. What problems, if any, would this man have in urinating?

CHAPTER 42

Control of Body Fluid Osmolality and Volume

Case 1: Gastroenteritis and Fluid Volume

A man weighing 60 kg (132 lbs) has an episode of gastroenteritis with vomiting and diarrhea. Over a 2-day period, this individual loses 4 kg (9 lbs) of body weight. Before he became ill, his plasma [Na$^+$] was 140 mEq/L, and it is unchanged by the illness.

Assuming the entire loss of body weight represents the loss of fluid, estimate the following:

Initial conditions (before gastroenteritis)

Total body water:	_____	L
ICF volume:	_____	L
ECF volume:	_____	L
Total body osmoles:	_____	mOsm
ICF osmoles:	_____	mOsm
ECF osmoles:	_____	mOsm

New equilibrium conditions (after gastroenteritis)

Total body water:	_____	L
ICF volume:	_____	L
ECF volume:	_____	L
Total body osmoles:	_____	mOsm
ICF osmoles:	_____	mOsm
ECF osmoles:	_____	mOsm

ICF, Intracellular fluid; *ECF*, extracellular fluid.

Case 2: Effects of Mannitol Infusion

A woman weighing 50 kg (110 lbs) and with a plasma [Na$^+$] of 145 mEq/L is infused with 5 g/kg (2.3 g/lb) of mannitol (molecular weight of mannitol is 182 g/mole).

Estimate the following equilibrium values. Assume that mannitol is restricted to the ECF compartment, that no excretion occurs, and that the infusion volume of the mannitol solution is negligible (total body water unchanged):

Initial conditions (before mannitol infusion)

Total body water:	_____	L
ICF volume:	_____	L
ECF volume:	_____	L
Total body osmoles:	_____	mOsm
ICF osmoles:	_____	mOsm
ECF osmoles:	_____	mOsm

New equilibrium conditions (after mannitol infusion)

Total body water:	_____	L
ICF volume:	_____	L
ECF volume:	_____	L
Total body osmoles:	_____	mOsm
ICF osmoles:	_____	mOsm
ECF osmoles:	_____	mOsm

Case 3: Renal Insufficiency and ADH

A patient with renal insufficiency has blood drawn, and the following values are obtained (normal values are indicated in parentheses):

Serum [Na$^+$]:	135 mEq/L	(140 to 145 mEq/L)
Serum [glucose]:	100 mg/dl	(90 to 100 mg/dl)
Serum [urea]:	100 mg/dl	(5 to 20 mg/dl)
P$_{osm}$:	310 mOsm/kg H$_2$O	(285 to 295 mOsm/kg H$_2$O)

Would you expect the plasma ADH levels in this individual to be elevated or suppressed?

Case 4: Gastroenteritis and Blood Volume

A 35-year-old man develops an acute episode of vomiting and diarrhea and loses 3 kg (7 lbs) in body weight over a 24-hour period. A blood sample shows that the plasma [Na$^+$] is normal at 145 mEq/L. Indicate whether the following parameters would be increased, decreased, or unchanged from what they were before this illness.

Plasma osmolality	_____
Effective circulating volume	_____
Plasma ADH levels	_____
Urine osmolality	_____
Sensation of thirst	_____

Case 5: Euvolemia

A 21-year-old woman is euvolemic and ingests a diet that contains 200 mEq/day of Na$^+$ on average. What would the Na$^+$ excretion rate of this woman be over a 24-hour period?

Case 6: Edema

A 55-year-old man with heart failure has developed edema. During the past 2 weeks, his weight has increased by 4 kg (9 lbs). Assuming that the entire weight gain is the result of the accumulation of fluid, calculate the following:

Volume of accumulated fluid	_____	L
Amount of Na$^+$ retained by the kidneys	_____	mEq

Case 7: Adrenocortical Adenoma—Hyperaldosteronism

In a 35-year-old woman an adenoma of her left adrenal gland produces high levels of aldosterone. This woman experiences retention of Na^+ by the kidneys (excretion < intake). However, after several days, Na^+ excretion increases to its previous level (excretion = intake). When the adenoma is surgically removed, Na^+ excretion increases (excretion > intake) but returns to its initial level over several days (excretion = intake).

1.   Delineate the mechanisms involved in these aldosterone-induced changes in Na^+ excretion.

Case 8: Myocardial Infarction and Renal Function

A 65-year-old man had a myocardial infarction 4 months ago, and now he complains of easy fatigability, shortness of breath, and swelling of his ankles. On physical examination he is found to have distended neck veins and pitting edema of the ankles. His breathing is rapid (20 respirations/min), and rales are heard bilaterally at the bases of the lungs. He is afebrile, his pulse rate is 90 beats/min, and his blood pressure is 110/70. Since his myocardial infarction, he has been taking a cardiac glycoside and a thiazide diuretic. A blood sample is obtained, and the following abnormalities are noted:

Serum $[Na^+]$	= 130 mEq/L	(normal: 135 to 147 mEq/L)
Serum $[K^+]$	= 3 mEq/L	(normal: 3.5 to 5 mEq/L)
Serum $[HCO_3^-]$	= 30 mEq/L	(normal: 22 to 28 mEq/L)
Serum [creatinine]	= 1.7 mg/dl	(normal: 0.6 to 1.2 mg/dl)

1.   Is the extracellular fluid (ECF) volume in this man above or below normal? What evidence in the physical examination supports your conclusion?

2.   Is the effective circulating volume (ECV) in this man above or below normal? What laboratory test could you perform to support your conclusion?

3.   How would you characterize renal Na^+ handling in this man? What evidence in the physical examination supports this conclusion?

4.   What is the mechanism for the development of hyponatremia in this man?

5.   What is the mechanism for the development of hypokalemia in this man?

6.   What type of acid-base disturbance does this man have? What is the mechanism for the development of this disorder?

7.   What is the significance of the elevated serum [creatinine]?

8.   The physician treating this man prescribes a loop diuretic in addition to the thiazide diuretic to further reduce his Na^+ retention and edema. What effect will this treatment have on the man's ECV? What is the potential effect of this treatment on the man's serum Na^+, K^+, HCO_3^-, and creatinine concentrations?

CHAPTER 43

Regulation of Potassium, Calcium, Magnesium, Phosphate, and Acid-Base Balance

Case 1: Acid-Base Disorders

In the following table, arterial pH and blood gas data are summarized for a number of patients with different acid-base disorders.

pH	$[HCO_3^-]$ (mEq/L)	PCO_2 (mm Hg)	Disorder
7.34	15	29	_____
7.49	35	48	_____
7.47	14	20	_____
7.34	31	60	_____
7.26	26	60	_____
7.62	20	20	_____
7.09	15	50	_____
7.40	15	25	_____

1. Indicate the type of acid-base disorder that exists for each patient. Use as normal values: pH = 7.40; $[HCO_3^-]$ = 24 mEq/L; and PCO_2 = 40 mm Hg.

Case 2: Gastroenteritis and Acid-Base Disorders

A previously healthy man develops a gastrointestinal illness with nausea and vomiting. After 12 hours of this illness, the laboratory data are shown in the table below. The illness continues, and after 60 hours the laboratory data are shown in the table below.

	12 hours	60 hours
Body weight:	70 kg	68 kg
Blood pressure:	120/80 mm Hg	80/40 mm Hg
Plasma pH:	7.48	7.5
PCO_2:	44 mm Hg	48 mm Hg
Plasma $[HCO_3^-]$:	32 mEq/L	36 mEq/L
Urine pH:	7.5	6

1. What is his acid-base disorder at 12 hours? What was its origin?

2. Has the acid-base disturbance changed after 60 hours? How do you explain the paradoxic decrease in urine pH?

Case 3: Glaucoma and Carbonic Anhydrase Inhibitors

A 50-year-old woman with glaucoma is treated with the carbonic anhydrase inhibitor acetazolamide.

1. What effect would administration of acetazolamide have on urine HCO_3^- excretion, and by what mechanism?
2. What type of acid-base disorder could result from the use of this drug?

Case 4: Diabetes Mellitus

A woman with insulin-dependent diabetes is given a β-adrenergic antagonist for treatment of hypertension.

1. If this woman was given an intravenous infusion of K^+, what would you predict would happen to the plasma $[K^+]$? Compare the response with a normal individual.

Case 5: Addison's Disease

A 49-year-old woman sees her physician because of weakness, easy fatigability, and loss of appetite. During the past month she has lost 7 kg (15 lb). On physical examination she is found to have hyperpigmentation, especially of the oral mucosal and gums. She is hypotensive, and her blood pressure (BP) falls when she assumes an upright posture (BP = 100/60 mm Hg supine, and 80/50 mm Hg erect). The following laboratory data are obtained:

Serum $[Na^+]$	= 130 mEq/L	(normal: 135 to 147 mEq/L)
Serum $[K^+]$	= 6.5 mEq/L	(normal: 3.5 to 5 mEq/L)
Serum $[HCO_3^-]$	= 20 mEq/L	(normal: 22 to 28 mEq/L)

1. The serum level of which hormone(s) would be expected to be below normal in this woman?

2. What is the cause of this woman's hypotension?

3. What is the mechanism for development of hyponatremia in this woman?

4. Why does this woman have hyperkalemia?

5. What is her acid-base disturbance, and what is the cause?

Case 6: Diabetic Ketoacidosis

An 18-year-old man with insulin-dependent diabetes mellitus (type I) is seen in the emergency room. He did not take his insulin during the previous 24 hours because he did not feel well and was not eating. He now complains of weakness, nausea, thirst, and frequent urination. On physical examination he is found to have deep and rapid respirations. At 2 AM the following laboratory data are obtained:

Serum $[Na^+]$	= 135 mEq/L	(normal: 135 to 147 mEq/L)
Serum $[K^+]$	= 8 mEq/L	(normal: 3.5 to 5 mEq/L)
Serum $[HCO_3^-]$	= 7 mEq/L	(normal: 22 to 28 mEq/L)
Blood pH	= 6.99	(normal: 7.35 to 7.45)
Arterial P_{CO_2}	= 30 mm Hg	(normal: 35 to 45 mm Hg)
Serum [glucose]	= 1200 mg/dl	(normal: 70 to 110 mg/dl)

The diagnosis of diabetic ketoacidosis is made, and the man is admitted to the hospital. Intravenous saline is administered, and insulin therapy is begun. At 3 AM, HCO_3^- is administered with more insulin. The results of therapy are illustrated below.

Time	Serum [K^+] (mEq/L)	Blood pH	Serum [HCO_3^-] (mEq/L)	Serum [glucose] (mg/dl)
2:00 AM	8	6.99	7	1200
3:00 AM	6	7.01	8	400
4:00 AM	4.5	7.1	12	100
5:00 AM	4.5	7.1	12	100
7:00 AM	3.5	7.08	11	100

1. What type of acid-base disorder does this man have?

2. Why did this man develop hyperkalemia?

3. Why did the serum [K^+] fall during the first hour of insulin infusion?

4. What effect will intravenous administration of HCO_3^- have on the serum [K^+]?

5. What is the mechanism for the polyuria in this man? What effect, if any, does the increased urine output have on his K^+ homeostasis?

6. This man's serum [Na^+] was 135 mEq/L before the initiation of therapy. By 7:00 AM it had risen to 152 mEq/L. What is the mechanism for the development of hypernatremia (i.e., increased serum [Na^+])?

THE ENDOCRINE SYSTEM

Saul M. Genuth

CHAPTER 44

General Principles of Endocrine Physiology

Growth Retardation in an Infant

A 6-month-old infant is evaluated for growth retardation. The pediatrician notes signs suggestive of deficiency of a peptide hormone. On further questioning, the pediatrician learns that one of seven siblings died in childhood with a similar clinical picture. A first cousin of the patient also exhibited this syndrome. Both parents, however, are apparently healthy. The pediatrician believes that an autosomal recessive genetic disorder causes this infant's apparent hormone deficiency state. The pediatrician uses knowledge of general endocrine pathways to investigate the possible causes.

1.   What three basic defects can you envision that would lead to the infant's hormone deficiency state?

2.   For each of these basic defects, what specific factors could be involved in this hormonal genetic disorder?

3.   How could you measure plasma or target cell samples to determine the precise endocrine lesion in this patient?

4.   What molecular biologic investigations would be required to prove your final diagnosis and to provide the basis for genetic counseling?

5.   Why don't all the siblings exhibit the biologic defect?

CHAPTER 45

Whole Body Metabolism

Starvation

A 26-year-old male prisoner begins a hunger strike to protest what he considers unfair prison policies. He drinks only tap water, and his only exercise is two daily half-hour walks at approximately 2.5 miles/hr. The temperature in his cell is maintained at 72° F. His starting weight is 70 kg (154 lbs), of which 14% is body fat. At the end of 4 weeks, he is urged by the prison physician, family, friends, and his attorney to stop his fast because of his deteriorating condition.

1. What would you estimate his daily energy expenditure to be?

2. Approximately how much weight would he have lost in 4 weeks? What would be the approximate distribution of this lost weight in carbohydrate, protein, and fat? In lean body mass and adipose tissue? What would his respiratory quotient be at that time?

3. What changes in plasma levels of energy substrates would occur in the first 3 days of his fast? What changes in urinary constituents would be expected?

4. On what immediate and on what ultimate sources of energy would brain metabolism depend?

5. What early changes in plasma levels of hormones would occur? How would this regulate his energy metabolism?

6. What other hormonal compensatory mechanisms would be called into play to conserve energy and prolong life?

7. What physiologic events would occur when he stopped his fast by drinking a large quantity of orange juice?

CHAPTER 46

Hormones of the Pancreatic Islets

Diabetic Acidosis

A 21-year-old brother of a person with insulin-dependent diabetes mellitus experienced increased urination and thirst for 6 weeks, along with a 15-lb weight loss, despite a normal appetite. Fearing that these symptoms meant he also had developed diabetes mellitus, he did not seek medical attention promptly. However, when he developed nausea and vomiting for 48 hours, followed by a stuporous state, his college roommate insisted on taking him to the emergency room. There, he was found to be semicoherent, and his mucous membranes and skin were dry. Blood pressure was 84/52 and pulse rate was 120 beats/min. He was breathing deeply at a rate of 30 respirations/min. The remainder of the examination was within normal limits. A urine sample contained a glucose concentration of 5% and tested strongly positive for acetoacetic acid. Plasma glucose was 800 mg/dl. Sodium was 132 mEq/L, bicarbonate was 5 mEq/L, chloride was 104 mEq/L, and potassium was 5.8 mEq/L. Blood pH was 7.1, P_{CO_2} was 17 mm Hg, and P_{O_2} was 95 mm Hg. Blood urea nitrogen was 28 mg/dl, and plasma creatinine was 1.4 mg/dl. On treatment with insulin, intravenous fluids, and potassium, the patient's clinical and biochemical status was restored to normal in 24 hours.

1. What is the cause of this patient's very high plasma glucose level?

2. What are the mechanisms that elevated plasma glucose?

3. Glucose production and release by the liver in part reflect the balance between glycolysis (glucose to pyruvate) and gluconeogenesis (pyruvate to glucose). What control points regulate the rates of bidirectional flow between glucose and pyruvate, and how are they affected by the relevant hormones?

4. What has replaced bicarbonate in the patient's plasma, and by what mechanisms?

5. Why is the patient breathing rapidly, and why is the blood pH low?

6. Why is the blood pressure low and the pulse rate high?

7. What levels of free fatty acids and triglycerides might you expect in plasma?

8. What levels of amino acids might you expect in plasma?

9. What other hormone levels would be increased in plasma?

10. What contributed to this patient's weight loss?

11. What caused his thirst and increased appetite?

12. What other constituents of the urine would be present in excessive quantities, especially when one considers that he had no food intake for 48 hours?

13. What effect would insulin treatment have on his plasma bicarbonate, pH, potassium, and phosphate levels?

CHAPTER 47

Endocrine Regulation of Calcium and Phosphate Metabolism

Parathyroid Adenoma with Renal Calculi

A 62-year-old man entered the emergency room with right flank pain. Urinalysis revealed hematuria, and x-ray studies demonstrated a stone in the right ureter. The stone was subsequently passed spontaneously, and analysis revealed it to be calcium oxalate. Further history disclosed two previous episodes of kidney stones, 10 and 20 years before. Recently, the patient had noted lethargy, polyuria, polydipsia, muscle weakness, and diffuse bone pain. Laboratory studies revealed the following levels: plasma calcium was 12.3 mg/dl, phosphate was 1.9 mg/dl, creatinine was 1.5 mg/dl, and albumin was 5.9 g/dl. Plasma alkaline phosphatase and urinary hydroxyproline were increased. Urinary calcium excretion was 380 mg/24 hr. After overnight water deprivation, urine osmolality did not exceed 290 mOsm/kg.

1. Is it certain that this patient has biologically significant hypercalcemia? How would you determine this?

2. What are the most likely hormonal causes of this patient's hypercalcemia?

3. For each hormonal cause, what are the mechanisms by which hypercalcemia is induced?

4. Which hormonal cause is most likely in view of the low plasma phosphate level?

5. For each hormonal cause, what would be the expected effect on the plasma levels of the other calcium regulatory hormones?

6. If hyperparathyroidism caused the patient's hypercalcemia, how would this explain the renal stones? Would a direct effect of parathyroid hormone (PTH) on the renal tubules be responsible?

7. If hyperparathyroidism were present, how would this explain the bone pain and the increases in alkaline phosphatase and urinary hydroxyproline?

8. Why did the patient have polyuria and exhibit inability to concentrate his urine? What would urinary cyclic AMP excretion be if he had hyperthyroidism?

9. When a single, very large parathyroid gland was surgically removed from the patient's neck, the serum calcium level might fall to 6 mg/dl. What two mechanisms would account for this? In each instance, what would you expect the plasma PTH and plasma phosphate levels to be?

10. If the patient hyperventilated when his plasma calcium level was low, what might occur?

CHAPTER 48

The Hypothalamus and Pituitary Gland

Case 1: Acromegaly

A 48-year-old man complaining of impotence sought medical attention. Over the years, he experienced increasing difficulty with maintaining and, more recently, achieving an erection. Further questioning revealed that he was also shaving less frequently. The patient's shoe size had increased from a 9-C to 11-EEE over the past 5 years, and his dental plate had to be altered three times in 6 years. Recently, friends have remarked on changes in his appearance. The patient also admitted to tingling of his fingers and joint pains.

On physical examination, he had coarse facial features with a bulbous nose and a beetle-browed look. The tongue was enlarged and teeth were wide spaced. Testing of visual fields showed a loss of both lateral (temporal) fields. The hands and feet were enlarged with spadelike fingers. The liver was enlarged. Laboratory studies showed a fasting plasma glucose level of 150 mg/dl. Fasting growth hormone (GH) was 40 ng/ml, and it did not decrease after administration of an oral glucose load. On magnetic resonance imaging, a large pituitary mass protruded upward from the sella turcica.

1. Why did the physician measure the GH?

2. The concentration of what other peptide is certainly elevated in this patient's plasma, and what is the source of this peptide?

3. What has caused the changes in the patient's facial features, tongue, hands, feet, and liver?

4. What has caused the neurologic and joint symptoms?

5. What is the normal effect of glucose administration on the plasma GH level, and why did it not change in this patient?

6. Why is the fasting plasma glucose level elevated, and what changes in the plasma insulin level would you expect to find?

7. What is the most likely cause of the patient's impotence, and what hormonal abnormalities explain it?

8. What effects might this pituitary tumor mass have on other anterior and posterior pituitary functions, and by what mechanisms?

9. What has caused the impairment of visual fields?

10. What molecule made in the hypothalamus might be therapeutically useful in this patient?

11. If the tumor mass were removed surgically, what physical changes would you expect to see in the patient?

12. If the normal anterior pituitary gland were removed surgically along with the tumor, what would be the consequences for the patient? How would you correct the situation?

13. If the patient wished to restore gonadal function, what hormonal replacement therapy would be needed?

Case 2: Diabetes Insipidus

A 30-year-old woman sustained multiple injuries, including a skull fracture, in an automobile accident. Although initially in a coma, she gradually regained consciousness. Five days later she abruptly developed frequent urination and thirst, with a subsequent measured fluid intake and output of 8 L/day. Physical examination was unremarkable except for slightly dry mucous membranes. Vital signs were normal. Routine urinalysis was normal; no red blood cells were present. Urine osmolality was 75 mOsm/kg. After 8 hours of water deprivation, during which she lost 4% of her body weight, she continued to excrete 150 ml/hr, and urine osmolality stabilized at 125 mOsm/kg. At this time, serum osmolality was 310 mOsm/kg, and serum sodium was 155 mEq/L. Serum creatinine was 0.8 mg/dl, and blood urea nitrogen was 10 mg/dl. There was no glucose in her urine.

1. What is the significance of this patient's urine osmolality being persistently less than plasma osmolality?

2. What is the significance of the elevated serum sodium level?

3. What portions of the nephron are critical to preventing excessive loss of free water, and what processes are involved?

4. What regulates the process of conserving free water, and how does the chief regulatory substance act on its target cells?

5. How and where is this regulatory substance synthesized and stored?

6. What modulates secretion of this substance?

7. What were the possible causes of this patient's polyuria and polydipsia?

8. What was this patient's plasma ADH level at the end of her water deprivation? Why?

9. What is likely to happen when ADH is administered to the patient?

10. What does the plasma ADH and the patient's response to ADH indicate about the diagnostic cause of her condition?

11. Assuming this patient's condition of polyuria and polydipsia is permanent, when would she need another dose of ADH?

12. What dietary components would influence the patient's urine output and how?

13. If the patient became stuporous again, what new dangers could arise despite continued treatment with ADH?

CHAPTER 49

The Thyroid Gland

Hyperthyroidism—Graves' Disease

A 34-year-old woman has a 3-month history of nervousness, tremor, palpitations, increased sweating, and discomfort with heat. She had lost 15 pounds despite increased food intake. She also noted muscle weakness and easy fatigability with exercise to which she was ordinarily accustomed. She had missed two consecutive menstrual periods. On physical examination, pulse was 110 beats/min at rest and rose to 150 beats/min with 30 seconds of rapid stair climbing. Blood pressure was 150/60 and respirations were 20/min. Her skin was warm and moist, her speech was rapid, her gaze had a stare quality, and her movements were hyperkinetic. She exhibited a tremor and very rapid reflexes, and she was unable to rise without assistance from a squatting position. The cardiac impulse was hyperdynamic, and the thyroid gland was diffusely enlarged. Laboratory studies showed a total serum T_4 level of 26 µg/dl (normal 5 to 12), a free T_4 of 4.1 ng/dl (normal 0.8 to 2.4), and a serum TSH of 0.01 mIU/ml (normal 0.5 to 5). A 24-hour uptake of radioactive iodine was 70% (normal 8% to 30%). A pregnancy test was negative. The patient was treated with a thiouracil drug. Four weeks later her symptoms had improved, and serum T_4 had decreased to 11 µg/dl. However, after 12 weeks of the same dose of the thiouracil drug, serum T_4 had decreased further to 4 µg/dl, and she complained of the recurrence of fatigue, lethargy, and intolerance to cold. Her weight had increased 20 pounds to a level above her usual healthy weight. Resting pulse was 54 beats/min. The thyroid gland, which had begun to decrease in size with drug treatment, had now grown even larger than before treatment.

1. By what mechanisms did an excess of thyroid hormone cause the various symptoms and physical findings this patient exhibited? How did her cardiac output and systemic vascular resistance compare with normal?

2. What genes may have been overexpressed or repressed by the high levels of thyroid hormone?

3. What was her serum level of triiodothyronine (T_3) likely to be and why? Would this contribute to her clinical state?

4. Why was her serum TSH so low?

5. Under what circumstances could her serum TSH have been elevated?

6. If her pregnancy test had been positive, how might this have affected her serum thyroid hormone levels?

7. What was the significance of her elevated radioactive iodine uptake?

8. What is the mechanism of action of the thiouracil drug?

9. What resulted at 12 weeks of therapy from continual exposure to the maximal dose of thiouracil drug?

10. What was her serum TSH level likely to be at that point and why?

11. Why did her thyroid gland reenlarge?

CHAPTER 50

The Adrenal Glands

Case 1: Adrenocortical Adenoma—Hyperaldosteronism

A 45-year-old man has a 10-year history of hypertension treated primarily with a thiazide diuretic. The patient had noted occasional bouts of muscle weakness and tingling sensations in his extremities. He denied vomiting. There was no history of pulmonary disease. Physical examination showed blood pressure (BP) of 158/102, pulse of 70 beats/min, and respirations of 6/min. Except for slightly decreased muscle strength, the examination was normal. There was no edema. Laboratory studies showed sodium of 146 mEq/L, bicarbonate of 35 mEq/L, chloride of 98 mEq/L, potassium of 2 mEq/L, creatinine of 0.9 mg/dl, blood urea nitrogen of 8 mg/dl, and fasting plasma glucose of 134 mg/dl. The diuretic was stopped, large doses of potassium were given orally, and an angiotensin converting enzyme inhibitor was prescribed for hypertension. One week later, BP was 154/98. Repeat laboratory studies showed sodium of 145 mEq/L, bicarbonate of 33 mEq/L, chloride of 98 mEq/L, and potassium of 2.6 mEq/L. After additional laboratory studies were performed, the angiotensin converting enzyme inhibitor was replaced with another drug, and potassium supplementation was continued. BP decreased to 130/82, and potassium increased to 4 mEq/L. The patient's symptoms disappeared.

1. What is the most likely acid-base disorder in this patient? What directional changes in pH and PCO_2 might you find in his arterial blood?

2. What are the possible causes of his acid-base disorder?

3. What evidence favors or casts doubt on each cause you have listed?

4. What urinary measurements would help define the cause of his problem?

5. What hormonal measurements would be helpful and in what physiologic state of the patient would you perform them?

6. How would increased secretion of a particular hormone have produced his hypokalemia?

7. What is the intracellular mechanism of action of this hormone?

8. What might explain the patient's muscle weakness and sensory disturbance? What electro-cardiographic effect might have been seen?

9. Why did the patient not have edema?

10. How could you explain the elevated fasting plasma glucose?

11. Why did the angiotensin converting enzyme inhibitor not lower the blood pressure very much?

12. What class of drug do you think the patient was given, and how did it work?

102

Case 2: Adrenocortical Adenoma—Hypercortisolism

A 48-year-old woman went to the local emergency room because of an abrupt onset of lower back pain. X-ray examination showed a compression fracture of the third lumbar vertebra along with evidence of osteoporosis in the spine. Further history revealed a 50-pound weight gain over the preceding 3 years, muscle weakness, and a tendency to bruise easily. She also complained of increasing emotional lability, including bouts of euphoria and depression. Sleep was also disturbed. Her previously regular menses were now only occurring every 4 to 6 months. Physical examination showed an obese woman with excess adipose tissue largely in the face, above the clavicles, and about the trunk. The extremities were thin and exhibited muscle atrophy. Skin was thin and had bruises that could not be accounted for by trauma. There were large purple marks over the abdomen. Excess hair growth was present on the upper lip and skin. Neurologic examination showed weakness of proximal muscle groups but normal deep tendon reflexes. Blood pressure was 164/102 and pulse was 76 beats/min. Laboratory findings showed fasting plasma glucose to be 180 mg/dl. Serum electrolytes showed a slight increase in the bicarbonate level and a slight decrease in the potassium level. White blood cell count was 16,000 with 92% neutrophils and 8% lymphocytes.

1. What is the most likely endocrine cause of this patient's clinical picture?

2. How would this hormonal disturbance produce the various symptoms and signs noted?

3. Why is the fasting plasma glucose level elevated? What would you expect the concurrent plasma insulin level to be?

4. What is responsible for the hypertension and slight abnormalities in the plasma levels of bicarbonate and potassium?

5. Why is there an excess of neutrophils and a deficit of lymphocytes in the patient's blood?

6. How would you establish the presence of the suspected hormonal hypersecretion?

7. What is the possible etiology of such hypersecretion?

8. How could you use the principle of negative feedback control to discriminate among the etiologic possibilities?

9. What other hormones are likely to be present in excess in this patient?

10. The primary locus of this patient's disease was eventually determined to be the gland from which the hormonal disturbance originated and surgical removal was carried out. Postoperatively, she noted satisfactory weight loss and the return of a normal emotional state. However, she also developed generalized weakness, lethargy, and loss of appetite. Blood pressure fell to 98/62. What is now wrong with the patient, and how has this come about?

CHAPTER 51

The Reproductive Glands

Case 1: Amenorrhea

A 18-year-old woman consulted a physician because of her failure to initiate menses. She had experienced normal breast development at age 12, but no pubic or axillary hair had ever appeared. Height was 5 ft, 6 inches, weight was 120 pounds, blood pressure was 110/70, and pulse 60 beats/min. General physical examination was normal and confirmed the presence of well-developed breasts. The external genitalia were those of a normal female. The vagina, however, ended in a blind pouch and no cervix was seen. Neither ovaries nor a uterus was felt. Within the inguinal areas, a 1.5 cm mass was felt on each side.

1. Could this individual have an XX sex chromosome karyotype? If so, what might the diagnosis be? What would be inconsistent with this diagnosis?

2. Could this individual have an XO sex chromosome karyotype? What would be inconsistent with this diagnosis?

3. Could this individual have an XY sex chromosome karyotype? If so, what diagnoses might explain her condition? What would be inconsistent with each of these possibilities?

4. What are the inguinal masses likely to look like histologically?

5. For each of the sex chromosome karyotypes listed above, what are the patient's plasma levels of estradiol, testosterone, LH, and FSH likely to be?

Case 2: Infertility

A 28-year-old woman has been unable to conceive a baby for 7 years. She has irregular menstrual cycles (22 to 36 days) and no physical complaints. Her husband has a normal sperm count, and the sperm have normal motility and morphology. She seeks investigation of their infertility. General physical examination is entirely normal. The external genitalia have a normal female pattern. A normal-sized uterus and ovaries are palpated. All of this is confirmed by ultrasound examination of the pelvis.

1. Thinking in physiologic sequence, what are the possible causes of this woman's failure to conceive?

2. What evidence could you seek to investigate each possible defect in the sequence that you have considered?

3. What treatment could you design to correct each physiologic defect?

ANSWERS TO CASE STUDY QUESTIONS

CHAPTER 1

1. The spherical shape of the patient's red blood cells (RBCs) would be expected to lead to greater osmotic fragility. When a normal RBC hemolyzes, it first swells to an approximately spherical shape. Any attempt to increase its volume beyond this point causes hemolysis because membranes cannot stretch appreciably (although they can bend). In hemolysis focal microscopic "breaks" in the membrane allow the internal contents of the RBC to equilibrate with the extracellular fluid. The patient's RBCs are already spherical, so they cannot first swell to become spherical when placed in a hypotonic solution. The spherocytes thus hemolyze more readily when put in hypotonic solutions. (See p. 12 in *Physiology* 3rd ed.)

2. A major way in which cells prevent osmotic lysis is by pumping Na^+ out of the cell by the Na^+, K^+-ATPase. The Na^+ gradient helps to counterbalance the osmotic gradient in the other direction because of intracellular impermeant substances and permeant ions that are in equilibrium across the membrane. When RBCs are incubated at 37° C, in the absence of substrates for producing energy, ATP levels in the cell decrease. Eventually the pumping rates of Na^+ and K^+ diminish. Na^+ leaking into the cell down its electrochemical gradient transfers osmotic equivalent to the RBC interior. This process leads to swelling, and ultimately to lysis, of the RBC. Because the patient's RBCs are three times more permeable to Na^+ than normal, the swelling and osmotic lysis occur more rapidly. Moreover, the hemolysis of the spherical RBCs occurs more readily than hemolysis of normal RBCs for the reasons discussed in the answer to question 1. (See pp. 31-33 in *Physiology* 3rd ed.)

3. The patient's RBCs are aided in resisting swelling and hemolysis by having an elevated level of Na^+, K^+-ATPase in their plasma membranes. Thus when Na^+ leaks into the cells at an elevated rate (compared with normal cells), it can be pumped back out of the cell at a similarly elevated rate by the greater number of Na^+, K^+-ATPase molecules. When the ATP level falls during incubation, the Na^+, K^+-ATPase is no longer able to keep up with Na^+ influx. Cell swelling and lysis result. Providing the RBCs with ATP and with glucose (from which the cells can make ATP) allows the Na^+, K^+-ATPase molecules to keep pumping Na^+ out of the cell at elevated rates that compensate for the elevated rate of Na^+ leak into the cell. In this way glucose and ATP help to prolong the time of incubation that the patient's cells can undergo before the onset of appreciable hemolysis. The ability of glucose and ATP to prevent an elevated rate of autohemolysis is one of the best diagnostic criteria of the disease known as *hereditary spherocytosis*. This criterion helps to distinguish hereditary spherocytosis from other microcytic anemias. (See p. 31 in *Physiology* 3rd ed.)

4. Flexibility of erythrocytes is required for them to deform sufficiently to pass through the narrow slit in the basement membrane that separates the splenic cords from the venous sinuses of the spleen. The patient's spherical RBCs are less deformable than normal discoidal RBCs. The patient's RBCs are thus retained in the splenic cords to a greater extent than normal. Response to this engorgement of splenic cords is believed to contribute to the splenomegaly observed in patients with hereditary spherocytosis. While the patient's RBCs are delayed in the splenic cords, they tend to deplete their glucose and then their ATP levels, which results in osmotic hemolysis by the mechanisms described earlier. Moreover, splenic macrophages engulf and destroy RBCs retained in the splenic cords. (See p. 329 in *Physiology* 3rd ed.)

5. These observations prove that there is no defect in the patient's spleen but rather that the defect is in the patient's RBCs. (See p. 329 in *Physiology* 3rd ed.)

6. The patient's decreased RBC life span, and the resultant anemia, are partially compensated by an increased rate of erythropoiesis. In a febrile illness, the rate of erythropoiesis is decreased, leading to transiently increased anemia. (See p. 332 in *Physiology* 3rd ed.)

7. A major contributor to the shortened life span of the patient's RBCs is the increased rate of destruction of RBCs in the patient's spleen, for the reasons discussed in the answer to question 4. Removing the patient's spleen dramatically prolongs the life of the average microspherocyte and thus leads to a marked improvement in the patient's anemia. (See p. 329 in *Physiology* 3rd ed.)

CHAPTER 2

1. The hyperkalemia with a concomitant decrease in the amount of K^+ in muscle cells suggests that the hyperkalemia is caused by K^+ efflux from the cells, but the cause of K^+ efflux is not known. Net K^+ efflux from muscle cells might occur because of diminished rate of K^+ accumulation by the Na^+, K^+-ATPase, or an increased rate of K^+ efflux from the cell, or a combination of both factors. The observation that Na^+, K^+-ATPase is normal does not completely rule out a malfunction of this protein during an attack. (See p. 31 in *Physiology* 3rd ed.)

2. Elevating extracellular K^+ and decreasing the intracellular level of K^+ would decrease the potassium equilibrium potential and thus decrease the magnitude of the resting membrane potential. (See pp. 33-35 in *Physiology* 3rd ed.)

3. The decreased magnitude of the resting membrane potential initially brings the muscle cells closer to threshold for firing an action potential. For this reason, spontaneous, small fluctuations in the resting membrane potential may reach threshold. This results in spontaneous action potentials and contractions of skeletal muscle cells and leads to the contractures experienced by the patient early in an attack. (See p. 38 in *Physiology* 3rd ed.)

4. Prolonged depolarization of the muscle cell plasma membrane will lead to *voltage inactivation* of Na^+ channels in the membrane, which will result in the muscle cell's being unable to fire an action potential. This is believed to be the cause of the paralytic phase of an attack and is supported by the observation that during the paralytic phase, the patient's skeletal muscle cells may be electrically inexcitable. (See p. 42 in *Physiology* 3rd ed.)

5. Insulin immediately and powerfully promotes the uptake of K^+ by cells and the extrusion of Na^+ from cells. Administration of insulin thus corrects the hyperkalemia, restores cellular K^+ levels toward normal, and causes the resting membrane potential for the affected skeletal muscle cells to become closer to the normal resting value. In this way insulin is believed to terminate an attack of contractures or paralysis in these patients. (See p. 785 in *Physiology* 3rd ed.)

6. Long-term administration of salbutamol, a β_2-agonist, increases the activity of the Na^+, K^+-ATPase in skeletal muscle cells. In this way, salbutamol administration leads to increased sequestration of K^+ in muscle cells. Apparently this helps to prevent the K^+ efflux that underlies episodes of hyperkalemia with resultant contractures that may be followed by periods of paralysis. (See p. 31 in *Physiology* 3rd ed.)

CHAPTER 3

1. The finding is consistent with depressed function of cutaneous sensory receptors or with a failure of the mechanism by which action potentials are conducted or generated in the sensory nerve fibers. (See pp. 122-125 in *Physiology* 3rd ed.)

2. The initial tingling and numbness are consistent with a malfunction of the cutaneous sensory system. The absence of superficial reflexes and the hypoactivity of deep reflexes suggest a more widespread failure of sensory input to and possibly motor output from the central nervous system. Finally, the patient's difficulty in walking, together with the other symptoms and findings, suggests a generalized deficit in action potential generation and/or conduction in the nervous system. (See pp. 122-125 and 198-204 in *Physiology* 3rd ed.)

3. The finding of a normal resting potential suggests that the resting K^+ conductance of the sensory nerve fiber is normal. The K^+ conductance is a major determinant of the resting membrane potential. Even a small change in the resting K^+ conductance would result in a proportional change in the resting membrane potential. This finding would also seem to rule out any major change in the resting Na^+ conductance. (See p. 34 in *Physiology* 3rd ed.)

4. The finding that the action potential evoked in the sensory fiber is slower to rise and of smaller height than normal, together with the fact that the resting potential is normal, suggests that there is a defect in the function of the Na^+ channels. If a smaller number of Na^+ channels than normal were participating in the action potential, a slower rate of rise and a smaller amplitude of the action potential would be expected. (See pp. 39-43 in *Physiology* 3rd ed.)

5. The delayed opening of K^+ channels and the voltage-inactivation of the Na^+ channels are the major determinants of the duration of the action potential. The finding that the action potential is of approximately normal duration suggests that there is nothing abnormal about the kinetics of opening of the K^+ channels and that the voltage dependence and time dependence of the inactivation of Na^+ channels are not abnormal. This, together with the reduced rate of rise and amplitude of the action potential, suggests that those Na^+ channels that are activated are functioning normally, but that a fraction of the Na^+ channels fails to open in response to membrane depolarization. (See pp. 39-43 and 48 in *Physiology* 3rd ed.)

6. The rapid onset (about 30 minutes) of the patient's symptoms, as well as the patient's neurologic deficits, are most consistent with a disorder known as *paralytic shellfish poisoning*. A toxin (saxitoxin) present in shellfish under some circumstances can cause these symptoms. Saxitoxin has actions similar to those of tetrodotoxin (the toxin from puffer fish). Saxitoxin blocks the opening of voltage-gated Na^+ channels in an all-or-none fashion. Saxitoxin is produced by certain dinoflagellates of the genus *Gonyaulax*. Shellfish that feed on these dinoflagellates concentrate the toxin in their tissues. When the dinoflagellates are abundant, they are responsible for the *red tide*, so-called because of reddish pigments they contain. Fishermen and public health officials have learned that shellfish should not be harvested during a bloom of these dinoflagellates, as indicated by a red tide. It is still not understood why the nerves and muscles of the shellfish are seemingly unaffected by levels of saxitoxin that are lethal to mammals. (See p. 374 in *Physiology* 3rd ed.)

7. Victims of paralytic shellfish poisoning sometimes die. When they do, it is because of paralysis of the respiratory muscles. After about 12 hours, if the victim has not experienced respiratory paralysis, the prognosis is quite good. Thus the patient should be monitored continuously for at least 12 hours so that mechanical ventilation can be established immediately should the patient cease breathing on her own. Typically, complete recovery from the symptoms of saxitoxin poisoning may require 24 hours or more. The slow recovery is the result of the extremely tight binding of the toxin to Na^+ channels (the dissociation constant is in the low nanomolar range). For this reason the toxin only slowly dissociates from the Na^+ channels so that it can be excreted in the urine. (See p. 374 in *Physiology* 3rd ed.)

CHAPTER 4

1. The simplest explanation of this result is that IgG from the patient blocks the voltage-dependent Ca^{++} channels of the adrenal chromaffin cell plasma membrane. These are the same type of voltage-gated Ca^{++} channels that are present in motor nerve terminals. (See p. 973 in *Physiology* 3rd ed.)

2. It appears that the block of the Ca^{++} channels by the IgG is all-or-none. This implies that the IgG acts to reduce the number of activatable Ca^{++} channels in the chromaffin cell plasma membrane (and by inference, in the motor nerve terminal). (See pp. 47 and 57 in *Physiology* 3rd ed.)

3. A major determinant of the frequency of mEPPs is the resting cytosolic Ca^{++} level in the motor nerve terminal. Thus the observation that the basal mEPP frequency is not affected by injecting IgG suggests that the IgG does not alter processes that set the level of Ca^{++} in the nerve terminal cytosol. In diaphragms from IgG-injected mice, the small increase in mEPP frequency in response to elevated extracellular K^+ is consistent with the explanation in answer 2. If the IgG reduces the number of voltage-activatable Ca^{++} channels, then fewer Ca^{++} channels will open in response to K^+-induced depolarization of nerve terminals in the diaphragm, the cytosolic Ca^{++} concentration in the nerve terminals will not rise so high in the IgG-treated diaphragm, and hence there will be a smaller increase in mEPP frequency in the IgG-treated diaphragm. (See pp. 56-58 in *Physiology* 3rd ed.)

4. The similar response of IgG-treated diaphragms and control diaphragms to the calcium ionophore suggests that it induces similar increases in intracellular Ca^{++} in the nerve terminals of the control and IgG-treated preparations and that the response to the elevated Ca^{++} is similar in both. This suggests that the IgG does not alter the events in the motor nerve terminal that occur after intracellular Ca^{++} rises. (See pp. 57 and 58 in *Physiology* 3rd ed.)

5. If the patient's IgG blocks voltage-dependent Ca^{++} channels in the motor nerve terminals, then an action potential in the motor neuron will release fewer quanta of acetylcholine; this will result in smaller EPPs. (See pp. 58 and 59 in *Physiology* 3rd ed.)

6. This blocking is best explained by assuming that the diminished size of the EPPs in the patient results in some EPPs not having sufficient strength to depolarize the muscle fiber to the threshold for firing an action potential. This hardly ever happens in a normal individual. (See p. 58 in *Physiology* 3rd ed.)

7. The likely explanation for the low-amplitude action potential is that some of the individual muscle fibers that are contributing to the compound action potential fail to fire action potentials in response to impulses in the motor axons that innervate them. As a result, fewer of the patient's muscle fibers will contribute to each compound muscle action potential. (See pp. 117 and 188 in *Physiology* 3rd ed.)

8. Following vigorous exercise, most of the nerve terminals in the muscle being studied have been activated at high frequency. For a period after the high-frequency stimulation, the motor nerve terminals will release more acetylcholine in response to a normal depolarization by the same processes that occur in post-tetanic potentiation. The cellular bases of post-tetanic potentiation are not completely understood. (See p. 66 in *Physiology* 3rd ed.)

9. *Plasmapheresis* will reduce the concentration of circulating antibodies that are blocking Ca^{++} channels and thus will increase the fraction of Ca^{++} channels in the prejunctional motor nerve terminals that behave normally. *Immunosuppressive therapy* should have the same effect. *4-Aminopyridine* will block voltage-gated K^+ in the motor nerve terminal. As a result, the depolarization of the nerve terminal

caused by the action potential will be prolonged. Thus activation of the voltage-dependent Ca^{++} channels will be prolonged. Influx of Ca^{++} into the nerve terminal will increase and thereby will release more acetylcholine. (See p. 42 in *Physiology* 3rd ed.)

CHAPTER 5

1. The patient has most likely taken in *Vibrio cholerae* in contaminated drinking water. In tropical countries without well-developed sewer systems, the flooding from monsoon rains frequently results in the contamination of drinking water sources with fecal bacteria such as *Vibrio cholerae*. This bacterium has colonized the patient's small intestine, where it releases a protein known as cholera toxin. Cholera toxin has two subunits. One cholera toxin subunit binds to GM_1 gangliosides on the luminal surface of the brush border plasma membrane of the small intestine and thereby provides a pathway for the other subunit of cholera toxin to enter the cell. The cholera toxin subunit that enters the cells is an enzyme that catalyzes the transfer of ADP-ribose to the α submit of G_S, the heterotrimeric G protein that stimulates adenylyl cyclase. The ADP-ribosylated G_S is permanently locked in the active conformation. The activated G_S then irreversibly activates adenylyl cyclase in the brush border plasma membrane of the patient's small intestine. This leads to a prolonged elevation of the level of cyclic AMP in the cytosol of the epithelial cells. The elevated cyclic AMP results in persistent activation of electrogenic Cl^- channels in the brush border plasma membrane. The efflux of Cl^- from the cytosol into the lumen of the small intestine drives the flow of Na^+ into the lumen. The osmotic effect of the Cl^- and Na^+ secretion into the lumen of the small intestine causes the secretion of water into the lumen of the small intestine. The amounts of Na^+, Cl^-, and water that enter the colon exceed by far the ability of the colon to absorb them, resulting in the marked diarrhea experienced by the patient. (See pp. 701-703, 727, and 728 in *Physiology* 3rd ed.)

2. The patient's almost comatose condition is caused by severe dehydration. Rehydration of the patient with intravenous isotonic NaCl improves the patient's fluid balance. (See p. 703 in *Physiology* 3rd ed.)

3. The oral rehydration solution is designed to both restore the patient's hydration and correct electrolyte imbalances caused by her profound and prolonged diarrhea. The patient has lost significant amounts of bicarbonate and potassium ions in her voluminous stool. For that reason bicarbonate and potassium are included in the oral rehydration solution. To help the patient to absorb water from the rehydration solution, and thus to aid in restoring her lost extracellular fluid volume, glucose and NaCl are included in the oral rehydration solution. The brush border transporter that uses the electrochemical potential difference of Na^+ to power the active uptake of glucose transports two Na^+ ions together with one glucose molecule into the intestinal epithelial cell. Because of this obligatory coupling between the uptake of Na^+ and glucose, the presence of Na^+ in the lumen promotes the uptake of glucose, and the presence of glucose enhances the uptake of Na^+ (and thus Cl^- to preserve electroneutrality). The absorption of these solutes, Na^+, Cl^-, and glucose, osmotically powers the absorption of water from the lumen of the small intestine into the blood. This helps to restore the patient's extracellular fluid volume. (See pp. 691, 698, and 703 in *Physiology* 3rd ed.)

4. Those intestinal epithelial cells that are affected by the cholera toxin have their adenylyl cyclase molecules irreversibly activated. This persists as long as the cells themselves do. For this reason, giving the patient an antibiotic to kill the *Vibrio cholerae* in her intestine, without also giving oral rehydration therapy, would not have saved this woman's life. If this patient with cholera is given no antibiotic, but is kept hydrated and in electrolyte balance with oral rehydration therapy, she will recover. The diarrhea will clear the *Vibrio cholerae* from her gastrointestinal tract. As the affected intestinal epithelial cells are exfoliated into the lumen, they will be replaced by new epithelial cells that differentiate from the crypts of Lieberkühn as they migrate up out of the crypts to repopulate the epithelial surface of the small intestine. These newly differentiated cells are not affected by the cholera toxin, their cyclic AMP levels are normal, and they will not secrete Cl^- and thus Na^+ and

water at abnormal rates. It takes approximately 3 to 4 days for the entire epithelium to be replaced in this way. The total recovery time will be a day or two longer than that because of the time required for the patient to restore her extracellular fluid volume and electrolyte composition to near normal levels. If the patient is kept hydrated and in reasonable electrolyte balance, normal physiologic processes will cure her of this disease. (See pp. 703 and 707 in *Physiology* 3rd ed.)

CHAPTER 6

1. The ventricles in this infant are dilated because the cerebrospinal fluid (CSF) produced by the choroid plexuses in the lateral, third, and fourth ventricles cannot escape rapidly enough into the subarachnoid space through the lateral and medial foramina (of Luschka and Magendie) in the roof of the fourth ventricle. The CSF pressure therefore builds up, and this causes dilatation of the ventricles. (See pp. 96-97 in *Physiology* 3rd ed.)

2. This type of hydrocephalus is noncommunicating, because the fluid communication between the ventricular system and the subarachnoid space is impaired. In communicating hydrocephalus, CSF drainage is impaired within the subarachnoid space or at the level of the arachnoid villi. (See p. 97 in *Physiology* 3rd ed.)

3. The obstruction in this case is likely to be caused by a malformation of the brainstem and cerebellum (Arnold-Chiari malformation), because other defects (spina bifida) in development of the nervous system are evident. Another possibility is absence or incomplete formation of the lateral and medial foramina (of Luschka and Magendie). (See p. 96 in *Physiology* 3rd ed.)

4. The CSF pressure that often exists in cases of infantile hydrocephalus is in the range of 200 mm H_2O. Normal CSF pressure in infants is around 40 to 90 mm H_2O. CSF pressure in adults is higher, 120 to 180 mm H_2O. (See p. 96 in *Physiology* 3rd ed.)

5. As the ventricles in hydrocephalus dilate, they will contain more CSF; thus the CSF volume is increasing. As long as the cranial sutures are still open, the increased volume of CSF can be contained within the skull without substantially reducing the brain and blood volumes. However, as the sutures close, brain tissue and its blood supply are compromised, and nervous tissue is lost. (See p. 97 in *Physiology* 3rd ed.)

6. Many untreated cases of infantile hydrocephalus are fatal during the first several years. Many of the survivors are mentally retarded and have various neurologic abnormalities. Surgically treated cases result in a much greater survival rate and mental capability than untreated cases. Although surgery may yield favorable results, there are also risks. As the patient grows, shunts around the obstruction require adjustment to accommodate the larger body size; this means additional surgical procedures. The shunt may become occluded or infected. In the case of peritoneal shunts (to peritoneal cavity) the catheter can perforate one of the viscera or disrupt the function of abdominal organs. (See p. 97 in *Physiology* 3rd ed.)

7. Hydrocephalus can occur also in adults. However, because the cranial sutures are closed, the head does not enlarge. Instead, the ventricles expand at the expense of brain and blood volume. Hydrocephalus in adults can be produced by a number of neurologic disorders, including tumors of the brain or pituitary gland, subarachnoid hemorrhage, and meningitis. Some cases of adult hydrocephalus are associated with normal CSF pressure (hydrocephalus ex vacuo). (See p. 97 in *Physiology* 3rd ed.)

8. Spina bifida may be relatively harmless if it simply represents a defect in closure of the vertebrae. However, meningocele or meningomyelocele may be associated. In the latter case, there may be weakness and atrophy of the leg muscles, sensory changes in the lower extremities, and urinary incontinence. Meningitis is also a danger. (See pp. 115, 122-127, and 253-254 in *Physiology* 3rd ed.)

CHAPTER 7

1. The weakness of the muscles in the distribution of the sciatic nerve was caused by the interruption of this nerve. The pattern of motor loss (weakness of the hamstring muscles, as well as of more distal muscles) indicates a proximal location of the interruption. A proximal location is consistent with the location of the gunshot wound in the thigh. The transection of the sciatic nerve interrupted sciatic nerve motor axons that originated from motoneurons in the ventral horn of the lumbosacral spinal cord. Therefore, motor commands could no longer reach the muscles supplied by the sciatic nerve, and hence the muscles could not longer be activated. (See p. 115 in *Physiology* 3rd ed.)

2. The sensory loss was caused by interruption of sensory axons in the sciatic nerve. The cutaneous sensory loss was in the distribution of the sciatic nerve. Sensory function in muscles and joints would also be lost. The cell bodies of the sensory neurons of the sciatic nerve are in dorsal root ganglia of the lumbosacral enlargement. (See pp. 93 and 109 in *Physiology* 3rd ed.)

3. Autonomic function in the distal part of the left leg would also be lost because the sciatic nerve contains sympathetic postganglionic axons, as well as somatic motor and sensory axons. (See pp. 93 and 244-247 in *Physiology* 3rd ed.)

4. Skeletal muscle fibers depend on innervation for their maintenance. Motor axons may release a trophic factor that provides signals to the muscle. Denervation deprives the muscle cells of this trophic factor, and it leads to their atrophy and eventual disappearance if the muscle is not reinnervated. Muscle that is not used will also atrophy to some extent ("disuse atrophy"), and this type of atrophy is not nearly as profound as denervation atrophy. (See p. 107 in *Physiology* 3rd ed.)

5. After complete denervation of a skeletal muscle, motor unit potentials can no longer be observed because these potentials depend on the synchronous activation of a collection of muscle fibers by an individual motor axon. The motor unit, which consists of a motoneuron and all of the muscle fibers that it innervates, is disrupted when the axons that connect the motoneuron cell body with the muscle fibers are severed. Fibrillations are spontaneous contractions of denervated individual muscle fibers. They are recognized in electromyography by their narrow and relatively small action potentials. Furthermore, they do not respond to attempts at voluntary contractions. Motor unit potentials are broader and larger because they represent the compound action potentials of many muscle fibers. Some asynchrony in the action potentials of different muscle fibers also occurs. (See pp. 115 and 118 in *Physiology* 3rd ed.)

6. After a motor axon is severed, several events occur. There are retrograde changes in the motoneuronal cell body (chromatolysis), and the axon distal to the lesion degenerates (Wallerian degeneration). Sprouts emerge from the distal end of the axon, and if these reach the distal part of the nerve, one of the sprouts will grow along a row of Schwann cells (band of Bungner). If this axon reaches its previous target muscle, it can reinnervate the muscle and restore its function; the rate of regeneration is about 1 mm/day. Naturally, the first muscles to regain function are those nearest the level of the injury. More distal muscles will recover at later times, provided that regenerating motor axons reach them before atrophy is complete. (See pp. 104 and 106 in *Physiology* 3rd ed.)

7. Recovery is incomplete because not all axons will reach their original target destinations. Some sprouts will grow in the wrong direction, others may form a neuroma (a tangled web of axonal sprouts, including sensory axons that may produce pain), and still others may follow the wrong row

of Schwann cells and innervate the wrong muscle or even other structures. Only reinnervation of the original target will restore normal function. (See p. 106 in *Physiology* 3rd ed.)

8.   Sensory axons regenerate in much the same way as motor axons, and so sensory function may recover as well as motor function. However, in some individuals nerve injury results in a chronic neuropathic pain syndrome. (See pp. 106 and 133 in *Physiology* 3rd ed.)

9.   Membrane components and cytoskeletal proteins needed for the regeneration of an axon are manufactured in the cell bodies of motor and sensory neurons. (See p. 99 in *Physiology* 3rd ed.)

10. Materials used for regrowth of axons are transported from the cell body along the axon by slow anterograde axonal transport. The rate of this transport is about 1 mm/day, which accounts for the rate of regeneration of the axons. (See pp. 103, 104, and 105 in *Physiology* 3rd ed.)

CHAPTER 8

Case 1

1. The spinal cord and perhaps some spinal roots were damaged. This is shown by prominent neurologic deficits that can only be explained by a central nervous system lesion. For example, a single spinal cord lesion can account for the loss of some sensations on one side of the body and of other sensations on the opposite side of the body. No such simple explanation is available to account for the clinical picture if the lesion only affected peripheral nerves. Furthermore, increases in stretch reflexes and the appearance of a Babinski sign result from interruption of central, but not peripheral, motor pathways. (See pp. 129-133, 213, and 219 in *Physiology* 3rd ed.)

2. The clue to the segmental level of the lesion is the distribution of the sensory loss. Pain and temperature were lost on the left side below the umbilicus. The dermatome in which the umbilicus lies is T10; that is, the sensory fibers that supply the skin in the region of the umbilicus enter the spinal cord over the T10 dorsal root. If a knife wound to the spine damages the T10 segment of the spinal cord, the knife will have entered the vertebral canal at about the level of the T7 or T8 vertebra. The reason for the segmental discrepancy between the vertebral column and the spinal cord is that the spinal cord stops elongating during development before the vertebral column does. (See pp. 94, 127, and 128 in *Physiology* 3rd ed.)

3. Nociceptive and thermoreceptive primary afferent fibers that supply the left lower trunk and lower extremity enter the spinal cord through dorsal roots below T10 (T11-S5) and synapse in the dorsal horn of the spinal cord. Activity in these sensory fibers activates spinothalamic tract cells at approximately the same levels. The axons of the spinothalamic tract cells cross to the other side and ascend to the brain in the anterolateral white matter of the right side of the spinal cord. If a knife wound on the right side at approximately the T10 level of the spinal cord hemisects the spinal cord, the wound would interrupt the spinothalamic tract on the right. Thus, it would prevent pain and temperature information that arises in the left lower trunk and lower limb from being signaled to the brain. (See pp. 131-133 in *Physiology* 3rd ed.)

4. The nervous system pathway that is responsible for vibratory sense is the dorsal column–medial lemniscus system. At the spinal cord level, the part of this system that carries sensory information from the lower extremity is the gracile fasciculus. Many of the axons in the gracile fasciculus are branches of primary afferent fibers that enter dorsal roots on the same side of the spinal cord and ascend to the medulla to synapse in the nucleus gracilis. Others belong to the postsynaptic dorsal column pathway, which originates from neurons in the dorsal horn. A knife wound on the right side that completely interrupts the gracile fasciculus will disrupt vibratory sensation that arises from levels below the lesion. In the cervical spinal cord, the equivalent pathway is the cuneate fasciculus. This pathway contains primary afferent and postsynaptic dorsal column axons that supply the upper extremity and upper trunk. However, the cuneate fasciculus differs from the gracile fasciculus in that it mediates both vibratory and position senses. The pathway from the lower extremity that is responsible for position sense travels in the gracile fasciculus only as far as the thoracic and upper lumbar spinal cord; here the axons from primary afferent fibers that signal position sense synapse in Clarke's column. Neurons in Clarke's column then project axons in the dorsal spinocerebellar tract, from which collaterals pass to a small relay nucleus in the medulla called nucleus Z. However, a knife wound that interrupts the dorsal spinal cord at a lower thoracic level will block both vibratory and position sense, because the axons of the afferent fibers of both pathways ascend in the lower part of the gracile fasciculus. (See pp. 129-131 in *Physiology* 3rd ed.)

5. The dorsal column–medial lemniscus pathway is responsible for discriminative touch. However, the spinothalamic tract also has a tactile function, although the resolution is less fine. Because the knife wound left the spinothalamic tract on the left side of the spinal cord intact, and because the left spinothalamic tract carries tactile information from the right side, there was no overt loss of touch on the right despite interruption of the right gracile fasciculus. However, careful sensory testing would reveal a loss of fine discrimination (such as the recognition of numbers traced on the digits). Vibratory sense is rarely tested on the trunk, and position sense cannot be tested on the trunk. (See pp. 129-133 in *Physiology* 3rd ed.)

6. Higher frequency vibrations are signaled by Pacinian corpuscles and position sense by muscle spindles. For distal joints, such as those of the fingers, a contribution to position sense is also made by Ruffini (SAII) receptors and joint receptors. (See pp. 122, 126, 127, and 198 in *Physiology* 3rd ed.)

7. The right lower extremity was paralyzed because the knife wound interrupted the lateral corticospinal tract, which is the main motor control pathway for voluntary movements. The lateral corticospinal tract that descends on the right side of the spinal cord originates from the left motor cortex. (See pp. 213-215 in *Physiology* 3rd ed.)

8. When a major part of the descending motor control systems is suddenly interrupted, as when the spinal cord is transected, spinal reflexes are generally reduced or lost for a period of 3 to 4 weeks. The causes of this "spinal shock" are unclear, but they presumably include a sudden loss of a descending tonic excitatory drive originating in the motor control centers of the brain. One proposed explanation for the later development of hyperactive stretch reflexes is sprouting of afferent nerve fibers to fill synapses vacated by degenerating descending motor fibers. (See p. 197 in *Physiology* 3rd ed.)

9. The sign of Babinski (extensor plantar response) may represent a primitive flexion reflex to noxious stimulation of the sole of the foot. It is normally present in infants, but becomes suppressed as the lateral corticospinal tract is myelinated and becomes functional. Interruption of the lateral corticospinal tract allows the reexpression of this flexion reflex. Under these conditions, the sign of Babinski is regarded as a pathologic reflex. (See p. 219 in *Physiology* 3rd ed.)

10. Although axons in the central nervous system can sprout and reestablish synaptic connections under certain circumstances, the success of regeneration in the central nervous system is much more restricted than that in the peripheral nervous system. A number of explanations for this have been proposed. However, an important possibility is that trophic substances needed to support regeneration may not be appropriately expressed (or inhibitory substances that interfere with regeneration may be expressed). (See pp. 106 and 107 in *Physiology* 3rd ed.)

Case 2

1. Morphine given systemically may act primarily at the level of the periaqueductal gray in the midbrain. This area is richly provided with opiate receptors, and microinjection of opiates here produces analgesia. The mechanism of the opiate action may reduce the activity of inhibitory interneurons, and the reduced activity may disinhibit the descending analgesia pathways that originate in the periaqueductal gray. These analgesia pathways in turn inhibit nociceptive transmission (e.g., by inhibiting spinothalamic tract neurons) in the spinal cord dorsal horn. (See pp. 138 and 139 in *Physiology* 3rd ed.)

2. Opiate receptors also occur in the spinal cord dorsal horn. For effective activation, these receptors require a higher dose of systemic morphine than do those in the periaqueductal gray. However, they can be directly activated if morphine is applied to the spinal cord. This can be done by epidural injection. (Morphine readily penetrates the dura because of its solubility in lipid membranes.) Thus epidural infusion of morphine can be used to block nociceptive transmission at the spinal cord level. Patient-controlled analgesia is becoming a widely accepted technique. In the usual hospital setting, morphine doses are given too infrequently to allow the plasma concentration to remain at a stable level. Thus the plasma concentration swings between a level that is insufficient for analgesia and one that causes somnolence. With patient control, the morphine level is kept optimal for analgesia. Interestingly, the total dose is less than that usually given with the alternative regimen. (See pp. 138 and 139 in *Physiology* 3rd ed.)

3. Respiratory depression is a potential complication of a morphine overdose, whether the morphine is given systemically or by epidural pump. The opiate receptor antagonist, naloxone, can be used to counteract the action of morphine. (See p. 139 in *Physiology* 3rd ed.)

4. Anterolateral cordotomy used to be the procedure of choice to control cancer pain, especially when the cancer was at a low segmental level. However, the original open procedure required surgical exposure of the spinal cord. More recently, percutaneous cordotomy has become feasible, so that lesions are made by inserting a needle through the intervertebral foramen between C1 and C2. This can be done in conscious patients. However, destructive procedures are now generally thought to be less desirable than the use of analgesics to control pain. In the case of pelvic cancer pain, there is the further disadvantage that the pain originates bilaterally; therefore a bilateral cordotomy would likely be required. Bilateral percutaneous cordotomies run the risk of interrupting the descending respiratory control pathways. (See pp. 133 and 601 in *Physiology* 3rd ed.)

5. Deep brain stimulation is an experimental procedure that is not used in ordinary practice. When it has been used experimentally to control cancer pain that results from the activation of peripheral nociceptors, the main target has been the periventricular gray (just rostral to the periaqueductal gray). Stimulation in the periaqueductal gray has the disadvantage that eye movements generally result. In addition, stimulation in this area can evoke a sensation of fear. The effectiveness of periventricular gray stimulation is controversial. (See pp. 138 and 139 in *Physiology* 3rd ed.)

CHAPTER 9

1. The enlargement of the hands, feet, and facial prominences is typical of acromegaly, which is caused by hyperactivity of the acidophil cells of the anterior pituitary gland. Hypersecretion may be caused by the development of an acidophil tumor. In younger individuals, whose normal bone growth has not been completed, a similar hyperactivity of the acidophils can produce pituitary gigantism. (See pp. 914, 919, and 920 in *Physiology* 3rd ed.)

2. The hormone involved is the growth hormone. (See p. 914 in *Physiology* 3rd ed.)

3. The visual field defect is called a bitemporal hemianopsia; that is, the defect is in both temporal visual fields (bitemporal), and blindness occurs in half of the visual field (hemianopsia). This visual defect should be distinguished from binasal hemianopsia, a rare condition in which the visual field defect is in the nasal half of the visual fields of both eyes, and from homonymous hemianopsia, a more common condition in which the defect is in corresponding halves of the visual fields of the two eyes (nasal visual field of one eye and temporal visual field of the other eye). (See p. 158 in *Physiology* 3rd ed.)

4. Visual field defects in both eyes can be produced by restricted lesions of the visual pathways; this occurs at pathway levels at which the nerve fibers that carry visual information from both eyes are close to each other. This level would be at the optic chiasm and more centrally. The axons of retinal ganglion cells in the nasal halves of the retinas project through the optic nerve and then cross in the optic chiasm to enter the contralateral optic tract. The axons of retinal ganglion cells in the temporal halves of the retinas do not cross, but instead they course from the optic nerve along the lateral aspect of the optic chiasm to enter the ipsilateral optic tract. Retinal ganglion cells in the nasal halves of the retinas are responsible for vision in the temporal visual fields (because light from a temporal visual field crosses through the lens and strikes the nasal half of the retina). Conversely, retinal ganglion cells in the temporal retinas signal images in the nasal visual fields. Damage to the middle of the optic chiasm, as can be produced by a pituitary tumor, can interrupt the crossing axons from the two nasal hemiretinas, thereby producing a bitemporal hemianopsia. Furthermore, the axons on the undersurface of the optic chiasm are from the lower retinas. Hence a pituitary tumor will disturb vision first in the superior temporal quadrants of the visual fields. Pressure on the lateral aspects of the optic chiasm can produce a binasal hemianopsia (e.g., because of bilateral aneurysms of the internal carotid arteries). Homonymous hemianopsias are produced by lesions of the optic tract, lateral geniculate nucleus, optic radiation, or visual cortex on one side.

    Because of the partial decussation of the visual pathway in the optic chiasm, the components of the visual pathway on one side behind the optic chiasm are responsible for vision in the contralateral visual field. Therefore a lesion that completely interrupts the visual pathway at this level will cause a visual field loss on the opposite side; for example, a lesion that interrupts the visual pathway on the left side behind the optic chiasms will cause a visual field loss in the nasal visual field of the left eye and of the temporal visual field of the right eye. Incomplete lesions may cause quadrantal visual field defects. These will also be homonymous (i.e., occupy the corresponding parts of the visual fields of both eyes). For example, a lesion that interrupts Meyer's loop in the left temporal lobe (which carries signals from the lower retinas) will result in a superior right homonymous quadrantanopsia. (See pp. 156-160 in *Physiology* 3rd ed.)

CHAPTER 10

1. Acoustic neurinomas are slowly growing tumors of Schwann cells of the eighth cranial nerve. As they enlarge, they can cause loss of function of adjacent cranial nerves and also damage the cerebellum and cerebellar peduncles. In this case, deficits occur in the function of several cranial nerves on the right side, including not only the cochlear and vestibular parts of the eighth nerve (see answers to questions 3 and 4), but also the trigeminal nerve (see answer to question 6), the abducens nerve (failure of the right eye to deviate to the right beyond the midline), the facial nerve (see answer to question 5), and the glossopharyngeal and vagus nerves (deviation of the soft palate to the left). The right cerebellum is also damaged (gait disorder and ataxia of the right arm). (See pp. 129, 134, 179, 189, 190, 211, 222, and 238 in *Physiology* 3rd ed.)

2. Large acoustic neurinomas (or other mass lesions) cause an increase in intracranial pressure. This distorts the meninges and therefore induces pain transmission in the trigeminal system and results in headaches. Papilledema or swelling of the optic nerve head is caused by compression of the venous drainage from the retina through veins that course in the optic nerve. This condition can cause blindness. Nausea often accompanies increases in intracranial pressure and may be caused by pressure on the brainstem. (See pp. 97, 129, and 150 in *Physiology* 3rd ed.)

3. The type of deafness is sensorineural. Conduction deafness is generally not complete. The Weber test is conducted by placing the stem of a vibrating tuning fork in contact with the midline of the forehead or on the vertex of the skull. Normally, the sound can be heard equally well in both ears. In conductive hearing loss, the sound is heard better in the defective ear, whereas in sensorineural hearing loss the sound is louder in the normal ear. The Rinne test determines if air or bone conduction is heard best. The stem of a vibrating tuning fork is placed on the mastoid process. When the sound is no longer heard, the tuning fork is removed from the bone, and the fork is brought close to the ear. Normally, the sound is still heard, indicating that air conduction is better than bone conduction. In conductive hearing loss, bone conduction is better than air conduction. The Rinne test was not very helpful in this case because the deafness was complete; in cases of a partial sensorineural hearing loss, the Rinne test is positive (i.e., hearing is best for air conduction). (See p. 179 in *Physiology* 3rd ed.)

4. The caloric test is used to examine vestibular function. When cold water is placed in the external auditory canal of one ear (with the head tilted back to bring the horizontal semicircular canals into the vertical plane), nystagmus will normally develop, and the fast phase of the nystagmus will be toward the opposite ear. Warm water will produce nystagmus with the fast phase toward the ear that is irrigated. In this case, no nystagmus was produced when a caloric test was done on the right side, because the vestibular part of the eighth cranial nerve was interrupted along with the acoustic part of the nerve. (See pp. 185 and 221 in *Physiology* 3rd ed.)

5. The acoustic neurinoma in this case caused a loss of function in the nearby facial, glossopharyngeal, and vagus nerves. The result was not only loss of the motor functions of these cranial nerves (paralysis of the right side of the face, including the levator of the eyelid, and weakness of the soft palate on the right), but also loss of taste on the right side of the tongue. The patient would not have noticed this loss of taste because substances in the mouth would have stimulated taste buds on the left side of the tongue. However, a loss of taste can be determined in a careful neurologic examination. (See pp. 189 and 190 in *Physiology* 3rd ed.)

6. General sensation was lost on the right side of the face and tongue because the tumor damaged the sensory portion of the right trigeminal nerve. (See p. 129 in *Physiology* 3rd ed.)

7. The gait disturbance and ataxia of the right arm were caused by compression by the tumor of the cerebellar peduncles and cerebellum on the right side. (See p. 238 in *Physiology* 3rd ed.)

CHAPTER 11

1. The olfactory pathway on the right side has been interrupted, causing a unilateral anosmia. (See pp. 194-195 in *Physiology* 3rd ed.)

2. Because the disease apparently progressed relatively slowly, there is a strong possibility that the underlying problem is a brain tumor. A massive lesion, such as a meningioma in the olfactory groove, could explain the anosmia, because it might well compress the olfactory tract. If the tumor grew further, it could also affect the left olfactory tract and cause bilateral anosmia. The headaches are likely to be secondary to an increased intracranial pressure. (See pp. 96-97 and 194-195 in *Physiology* 3rd ed.)

3. The central scotoma in the right eye is caused by pressure on the right optic nerve, which passes close to the olfactory tract en route to the optic chiasm. Many axons of the right optic nerve must have been interrupted to cause the optic disc to become pale after Wallerian degeneration, with the consequent loss of myelin. (See pp. 106, 141-142, and 158 in *Physiology* 3rd ed.)

4. The changes observed in the left eye are typical of papilledema. This condition can result from an increase in intracranial pressure. The pressure is transmitted directly through the cerebrospinal fluid in the subarachnoid space to the optic disc; this occurs because the optic nerves are ensheathed by the meninges and are surrounded by a subarachnoid space at their origin from the optic disc. Pressure here will tend to cause venous stasis and edema in the optic nerve head. (See pp. 96-97, 141-142, and 473-475 in *Physiology* 3rd ed.)

5. If the lesion is an olfactory groove meningioma, this type of brain tumor can often be cured by surgical removal. However, it is unlikely that the patient will recover from the deficit in olfaction or the central scotoma, because axons in the affected neural structures have already been permanently lost.

CHAPTER 12

1. The trauma of the car accident functionally transected the spinal cord at the level of the neck. The segmental level of the spinal injury is suggested by the pattern of loss of voluntary motor control. The patient eventually had some motor function in the shoulder. Shoulder muscles receive a motor supply from the C5 spinal segment. The muscles that receive motor axons from the remainder of the cervical enlargement, C6-T1, are paralyzed; therefore the transection must have been at the C5-C6 level. (See p. 115 in *Physiology* 3rd ed.)

2. The patient could not move his extremities voluntarily because the descending motor pathways, including the corticospinal tracts, had been severed. (See pp. 197, 213-217, and 220 in *Physiology* 3rd ed.)

3. The patient could not feel anything below the level of transection because the somatosensory pathways, including the dorsal columns and the spinothalamic tracts, had been interrupted. (See pp. 129-133 in *Physiology* 3rd ed.)

4. The type of paralysis that results from the interruption of the corticospinal and associated motor tracts is known as a spastic paralysis. In normal individuals, phasic stretch reflexes can be elicited by tapping the tendon of a muscle, such as the quadriceps, to stretch the muscle and activate group Ia muscle spindle afferent fibers. The burst discharges of these stretch receptors cause synchronous discharges of alpha motoneurons that supply the same and synergistic muscles. Hence a tendon tap results in a contraction of the muscle whose tendon is tapped. In spastic paralysis, the motor control circuits in the spinal cord are altered (this is poorly understood). Therefore, gamma motoneurons become hyperactive, and their activity results in a greater sensitivity of muscle spindles to muscle stretches, especially to phasic stretches. Thus the phasic stretch reflexes become more active. Although muscle tone is increased, the most prominent change in spastic paralysis is the increase in phasic stretch reflexes. This change accounts for the appearance of clonus. When a muscle, such as the triceps surae, is stretched briskly by dorsiflexion of the foot, the contraction of this muscle causes plantar flexion of the ankle. This in turn stretches the pretibial flexors and elicits their contraction. This contraction stretches the triceps surae muscles once more (or the continued upward pressure on the foot by the examiner causes another stretch of the triceps surae), and causes another contraction. The result is a continued series of alternating contractions of antagonistic muscle groups and the consequent alternating movements of the ankle. (See pp. 198-205 and 219 in *Physiology* 3rd ed.)

5. The flexor withdrawal reflex becomes exaggerated below the level of a spinal cord transection because of interruption of pathways that descend from the brain and that normally tend to suppress the flexion reflex. These descending control systems include a pathway that originates in the medulla. (See pp. 197 and 205-207 in *Physiology* 3rd ed.)

6. After a spinal cord transection, the bladder initially becomes flaccid. At this time, urine retention becomes a major problem, and bladder infections are common. As spasticity develops, the bladder wall develops excessive tone, the bladder contracts reflexly or at irregular intervals, and incontinence develops. Evacuation of the bladder is still incomplete, and the bladder remains susceptible to infections. (See pp. 197 and 254 in *Physiology* 3rd ed.)

CHAPTER 13

1. The patient has had a cerebrovascular accident or "stroke" secondary to atherosclerosis accelerated by hypertension. (See pp. 461-462 in *Physiology* 3rd ed.)

2. The stroke was probably caused by thrombosis of an artery that supplied the region of the internal capsule on the left side. A large lesion of the left internal capsule can result in paralysis of the right lower face, arm, and leg. The voluntary motor pathways that control the right side of the body originate in the left frontal lobe, and they pass through the internal capsule on the left side. They cross to the opposite side at the junction of the medulla with the spinal cord. The damage probably was not restricted to the cortical level, because the widespread loss of motor function would imply a very large cortical lesion that would include the face, arm, and leg areas of the motor cortex. (See pp. 214-219 and 225-229 in *Physiology* 3rd ed.)

3. The motor pathways that were interrupted included the corticospinal and corticobulbar tracts and the associated corticoreticular and other brainstem projections. A pure lesion of the corticospinal tract results in a flaccid paralysis. Presumably, the interruption of the associated motor pathways causes the paralysis to be spastic. The patient could wrinkle her brow and close her eyes, yet she had paralysis of her lower face because of the organization of the corticobulbar control of the facial nucleus. Facial motoneurons that supply the muscles of the upper face receive a bilateral corticobulbar supply. Thus a lesion that interrupts the corticobulbar tract on one side will not paralyze these muscles. However, the motoneurons of the facial nucleus that supply the lower face receive only a contralateral input from the motor cortex; therefore if this input is interrupted, the lower face is paralyzed. (See p. 219 in *Physiology* 3rd ed.)

4. The speech problem of the patient is a type of aphasia. Dysarthria (faulty speech because of difficulty in performing the movements needed for speech) may result from lesions of the corticobulbar tract, but in this case the patient did not speak at all. Because the patient could understand the physician's directions (e.g., the request to raise the right arm), the patient did not have a receptive aphasia. Instead, the aphasia was expressive. Such aphasias are generally attributed to damage of Broca's area in the inferior frontal gyrus of the dominant hemisphere (which is usually the left hemisphere). In this case, it is unclear if the aphasia resulted from interruption of the pathways connecting Broca's area to other parts of the brain or if Broca's area was damaged, as well as the internal capsule. (See p. 271 in *Physiology* 3rd ed.)

5. The patient could have several types of sensory deficit. Interruption of the internal capsule can disconnect the somatosensory thalamus from the sensory cortex and thereby cause a loss of somatic sensation. This will be especially severe with respect to tactile discrimination, vibratory sense, and position sense, with less effect on pain. This is true because the dorsal column–medial lemniscus system depends more on the SI cortex than on the spinothalamic system. If the large capsular lesion extends far enough posteriorly, it could interrupt the optic radiation and produce a right homonymous hemianopsia. (See pp. 134-137 and 157 in *Physiology* 3rd ed.)

CHAPTER 14

Case 1

1. The patient had lesions in several distinct parts of the nervous system. For example, before the present illness, she had a visual deficit. She had a central scotoma that must have been caused by a lesion in either the left optic nerve, the optic nerve head, or the retina. The pale left optic disc is the result of demyelination of optic nerve fibers. She now has signs of a motor disorder. Furthermore, she has a history of acute episodes of a variety of neurologic disorders that underwent remission after a short time. The clinical picture is typical of multiple sclerosis. (See p. 158 in *Physiology* 3rd ed.)

2. The ataxic gait, nystagmus, intention tremor, and dysdiadochokinesia can all be ascribed to cerebellar damage. However, it is possible that other structures, such as the vestibular system and spinal cord, are also involved. (See pp. 233-234 and 238-239 in *Physiology* 3rd ed.)

3. The phasic stretch reflexes observed in cerebellar disease are often "pendular." For example, when the patellar tendon is struck by a reflex hammer, the knee jerk is followed by a series of oscillations of the leg. In contrast to clonus, these movements are associated with a reduction in muscle tone and are caused by failure of stretch reflexes in the antagonistic muscles to dampen the movement induced by the initial reflex. (See p. 239 in *Physiology* 3rd ed.)

Case 2

1. The tremor of Parkinson's disease is a tremor at rest; that is, it is worse when the person is in repose, and it gets better when the person is using his hands. The cerebellar intention tremor is really a manifestation of incoordination, and it appears when the person is actively using a limb. (See pp. 238-239 and 242 in *Physiology* 3rd ed.)

2. Characteristic of Parkinson's disease, besides the tremor, are rigidity and bradykinesia. The muscles remain partially contracted, and when a joint is passively bent, considerable resistance is felt by the examiner. As the joint bends, sudden catches are felt; hence the name "cog-wheel" is applied to this form of rigidity. The bradykinesia is presumably attributable to the patient's difficulty in moving because of the rigidity. Curiously, the phasic stretch reflexes are not changed in any predictable way. Therefore increased excitability of muscle spindles is probably not responsible for the increased muscle tone. The alpha motoneurons may be excited directly by descending motor commands. Alternatively, the static gamma motoneurons may be most affected. (See pp. 202 and 242 in *Physiology* 3rd ed.)

3. In Parkinson's disease, dopaminergic neurons in the substantia nigra are lost as also are neurons in other monoaminergic nuclei, such as the locus coeruleus and the raphe nuclei). The removal of dopaminergic terminals from the striatum may be the primary deficit. Therefore, neurons in the motor thalamus would be disinhibited, and hence activity in the motor cortex would be increased. (See pp. 239-242 in *Physiology* 3rd ed.)

CHAPTER 15

1. The unusual distribution of pain and temperature loss indicates that the lesion was in the dorsolateral medulla. This loss is caused by interruption of the spinal tract of the trigeminal nerve and by damage to the spinothalamic tract in the lateral medulla secondary to a cerebrovascular accident. Most commonly, this clinical picture results from occlusion of the posterioinferior cerebellar artery. (See pp. 131-134 in *Physiology* 3rd ed.)

2. The patient has Horner's syndrome. The symptoms includes a slight ptosis (drooping of the eyelid caused by paralysis of the superior tarsal muscle), miosis (constriction of the pupil), and anhidrosis (lack of sweating) on one side of the face. Horner's syndrome is caused by interruption of the sympathetic supply of the face. Often the interruption is at the level of the upper thoracic spinal cord or in the ascending sympathetic trunk. However, in this case it is caused by interruption of descending excitatory pathways that tonically activate the sympathetic outflow. (See p. 252 in *Physiology* 3rd ed.)

3. The motor disorder of this type involves an ataxic gait that is not made worse by closing the eyes, and it is most likely caused by damage to the cerebellum. The hoarseness would have been produced by damage to the nucleus ambiguus or its emerging motor fibers as they joined the vagus nerve. This damage would paralyze the vocal cords on one side. (See p. 238 in *Physiology* 3rd ed.)

CHAPTER 16

Case 1

1. The symptoms of narcolepsy resemble several of the features of rapid eye movement (REM) sleep. A person in REM sleep is very difficult to arouse. Sleep seems to be an overwhelming urge to the narcoleptic. The urge occurs even under conditions that can be life threatening, such as while he is driving a car on a freeway. In REM sleep, muscle tone is generally reduced. This parallels the bouts of cataplexy and also the sleep paralysis that occurs in narcolepsy. Finally, dreams occur primarily in REM sleep, and hypnogogic hallucinations occur in narcolepsy. (See p. 269 in *Physiology* 3rd ed.)

2. The electroencephalogram (EEG) during the sleep attacks of narcoleptics resembles that of REM sleep; that is, the EEG is of the low-voltage, high-frequency type. (See p. 269 in *Physiology* 3rd ed.)

3. Arousal is a function of the reticular activating system. Stimulant drugs, like the amphetamines, increase the activity of the reticular activating system. (See p. 270 in *Physiology* 3rd ed.)

Case 2

1. The seizure began as a partial focal motor seizure (Jacksonian seizure) that became generalized. The two types of generalized seizures are petit mal and grand mal. The patient's seizure was the grand mal type. Petit mal seizures are characterized by transient "absences" and not by tonic and clonic muscle contractions and the other manifestations shown by this patient. (See p. 270 in *Physiology* 3rd ed.)

2. The initial movements were characteristic of seizures that begin in the motor cortex and spread from a particular somatotopic site, such as the face area, to adjacent areas, such as the hand area. This progression is called a Jacksonian march, after the neurologist John Hughlings Jackson who described them. (See pp. 215 and 270 in *Physiology* 3rd ed.)

3. If the electroencephalogram (EEG) could have been taken during the seizure, there would have been a fast rhythmic activity during the tonic component and a series of slower large waves during the clonic phase. (See p. 270 in *Physiology* 3rd ed.)

4. The neurophysiologic basis for epilepsy has been investigated intensively for many years. Some epileptics have interictal spikes, which are EEG waves that occur between seizures. These shifts seem to represent summed depolarization shifts that can occur in individual cortical neurons in experimental models of epilepsy. The cause of these depolarization shifts is unclear, but they may result in part from the loss of inhibitory inputs that normally restrain the excitability of cortical neurons. A major inhibitory neurotransmitter in the cerebral cortex is gamma-aminobutyric acid (GABA); penicillin, a GABA antagonist, can cause seizures when it is experimentally applied to the cortex. (See p. 271 in *Physiology* 3rd ed.)

CHAPTER 17

1. Almost anyone who "overuses" a muscle (i.e., undertakes activity that leads to intense or sustained periods of force development) is likely to experience DOMS. The intensity of effort (magnitude of forces involved) seems to be more important than the duration of the effort.

2. The forces imposed on the muscle by gravity would be higher because attached crossbridges can bear a load some 1.6 times greater than the force that they can develop. Thus the forces on the contracting motor units of the left quadriceps muscle and its tendons would be greater than the forces in the contralateral muscle. (See pp. 288-290 in *Physiology* 3rd ed.)

3. This is unlikely because stretch of a contracting muscle does not result in ATP hydrolysis by crossbridge cycling. One might expect that glycogen depletion or some other factor that compromises ATP production, and thereby contraction, would be most pronounced in the right quadriceps, which has had a high metabolic rate during the exercise. (See pp. 296 and 304-305 in *Physiology* 3rd ed.)

4. This seems unlikely because the metabolism of the right quadriceps muscle would have been much higher than that of the left. Furthermore, although metabolite accumulation might contribute to temporary fatigue in voluntary contractions, no voluntary exercise induces cellular fatigue that would reduce the response to percutaneous stimulation. In addition, metabolic homeostasis is quickly restored, whereas the soreness and stiffness are not evident for many hours. (See pp. 304-305 in *Physiology* 3rd ed.)

5. The efficiency of chemomechanical transduction by crossbridges is estimated to be some 40% to 45% at most. Thus over half of the energy liberated during ATP hydrolysis appears as heat. The rise in temperature results from the inability of the circulation to remove the heat at the same rate that it is generated in a muscle. The absence of DOMS in the shortening right quadriceps, with its high rate of ATP consumption, rules out heat injury as a causative factor. (See pp. 288 and 296 in *Physiology* 3rd ed.)

6. Elevated serum creatine kinase and myoglobin levels must reflect muscle cell injury that allows leakage of these proteins from cells. The biopsy tissue samples provide further support for focal injuries in the sore muscle. (See pp. 300-301 in *Physiology* 3rd ed.)

7. In the absence of trauma, injury must reflect the imposition of forces that exceed the structural capacity of the affected cells to resist those forces. The highest forces in muscle cells occur when contracting cells are forcibly lengthened by imposed loads that result in negative work. Negative work is a normal part of muscle function, but it may cause injury in cells not regularly used in this way. (See pp. 306-307 in *Physiology* 3rd ed.)

8. The cells are very adaptable and respond to use by hypertrophy and perhaps by cytoskeletal and extracellular connective tissue alterations that enable the cells not only to develop higher forces but also to withstand higher imposed loads. The safety factor is not great, and regular exercise is needed to maintain the capacity to deal with high forces without injury. (See pp. 305-307 in *Physiology* 3rd ed.)

9. Pain as a signal to cease exercise in order to limit injury must be immediate. Thus no benefits for DOMS are evident except those that underlie the motivational "no pain, no gain" philosophy of athletes. (See pp. 125-127 and 133 in *Physiology* 3rd ed.)

10. The sensation of pain depends on activation of afferent nerve fibers. Because the onset of pain roughly parallels the rise in serum creatine kinase and myoglobin, it seems likely that dying or injured cells release agents that can activate the pain receptors. Such factors could include serotonin, histamine, K^+, pressure associated with edema, or inflammatory processes. (See pp. 964-966 in *Physiology* 3rd ed.)

CHAPTER 18

Case 1

1. The heart is a pump. All cardiac cells contract in synchrony in a prolonged twitch (heartbeat). The force and frequency of the heartbeat are physiologically regulated to adjust cardiac output to metabolic needs. The heart is continuously active and does not fatigue, although it is absolutely dependent on the maintenance of oxidative metabolism. Skeletal muscles are composed of independent fast and slow motor units that rarely contract in synchrony. Force is varied by recruitment of more motor units and tetanization. Skeletal muscles exhibit fatigue, with fast glycolytic (type I) motor units unable to maintain continuous activity. Arguably skeletal muscle could not substitute for cardiac muscle; however, as indicated in the case study, a conditioned skeletal muscle has some potential to assist a weakened heart. (See pp. 296-301, 304, 376-379, and 405-408 in *Physiology* 3rd ed.)

2. No, for the following reasons. (1) The heart still has its normal mechanisms to adjust its frequency of contraction. Therefore, the stimulator must be modified so that it is triggered by the endogenous cardiac cycle to synchronize contraction of the myocardium and the skeletal muscle. (2) Skeletal muscle twitches are brief and produce relatively low forces compared with cardiac systole. A practical cardiomyostimulator must generate bursts of action potentials to induce brief tetani matched to the ventricular systole. (3) Action potentials are not propagated from one skeletal muscle cell to another, and there is no pacemaker region in the latissimus dorsi. The stimulating electrodes of a cardiomyostimulator must be placed so as to stimulate most of the motor nerves to the motor units of the skeletal muscle. (See pp. 295 and 398 in *Physiology* 3rd ed.)

3. Some 4 to 6 weeks of progressive training by low-frequency electrical stimulation transforms fast, glycolytic motor units to slow, oxidative motor units that express the slow twitch isoform of myosin. The oxidative capacity of most type I slow motor units would be increased. In practice, sufficient resistance to fatigue can occur for indefinite pacing at normal heart rates. (See pp. 306 and 307 in *Physiology* 3rd ed.)

4. Some loss of collateral circulation is an inevitable consequence of such surgery, and an increased vascularization is necessary to meet the oxidative metabolic demands associated with continuous activity in all motor units. Considerable neovascularization and revascularization occur during adaptation. (See pp. 520 and 536 in *Physiology* 3rd ed.)

5. It is unlikely that sarcomeres would be much longer, because that would require stretching the muscle against the passive elasticity of the connective tissue and compression of the ventricles during diastole. The surgeon carefully avoids this because it would interfere with cardiac filling. However, it is inevitable that many fibers will be shortened as a result of the radical changes in geometry caused by surgery. The muscles adapt by removing sarcomeres at the ends of cells to shorten the cells and restore optimal sarcomere lengths. The mechanisms governing the addition or removal of sarcomeres are unknown. (See pp. 289, 305, and 306 in *Physiology* 3rd ed.)

6. The muscle may not generate large forces because studies suggest that this operation does not produce high stroke volumes or ejection fractions. Note, however, that the heart is a thick-walled organ. Hence it would not require a large amount of shortening of the latissimus dorsi to greatly reduce the volume of the ventricles. (See pp. 289 and 316 in *Physiology* 3rd ed.)

7.   Although striated muscle cells can hypertrophy in response to increased loads, they have a very limited regenerative capacity, in contrast to smooth muscle. (See pp. 306, 322, and 536 in *Physiology* 3rd ed.)

8.   There is no clear answer, but some factors to consider include the following. (1) This is still an experimental procedure, and improvements can be expected with further research. Although technical success has been achieved, there is no hard evidence for major improvements in cardiac function. (2) The procedure avoids the problems of tissue rejection, cardiac denervation, and sustained ischemia. (3) The technique is not suited for terminally ill patients, because of both the extent of the surgery and the prolonged time required to condition the muscle. (4) Because the pacemaker can be driven by the heart's own pacemaker region, it is theoretically possible to provide a better match between cardiac output and metabolic needs than with a transplant. (5) The procedure provides a dramatic example of the capacity of skeletal muscle fibers to adapt to activity patterns. Nevertheless, the special characteristics of muscle in hollow organs, such as mechanically and electrically coupled cells, are never achieved. (See pp. 305-307, 309, and 378-379 in *Physiology* 3rd ed.)

9.   Because all the original neural circuitry is preserved, it is likely that motor units are recruited inappropriately for assisting cardiac function. Factors that may minimize resistance to cardiac filling include the following: (1) most skeletal muscle actions involve only part of the motor units and they act asynchronously, so the forces might be low; (2) the electrical pacing at the heart rate frequencies will induce antidromic action potentials that will block normal action potentials elicited at the motor nerve cell bodies in the spinal cord; and (3) some learning process presumably takes place for appropriate use of the remaining muscles acting on the humerus to perform an act; this replaces motor unit activation in the left latissimus dorsi. (See pp. 114-118, 207-209, 225-228, and 301-303 in *Physiology* 3rd ed.)

10.   This would mimic the effects of activation of muscle spindles, Golgi tendon organs, and nociceptive nerves. The muscle spindles would contribute to reflex activation of the left latissimus dorsi and influence the recruitment of motor units in other muscles. The nociceptive nerves would induce the sensation of pain. The practicality of the procedure depends on the capacity of the nervous system to adapt, so that the conscious perception of pain disappears and functionally adaptive recruitment of motor units is reestablished. (See pp. 125-127, 138-139, and 198-209 in *Physiology* 3rd ed.)

Case 2

1.   Life without motion is impossible, and movement is generated by contraction of muscle cells. Locomotion, communication, respiration, eating, and many other activities that are needed to maintain life and that are essential to the quality of life depend on normal muscle function. (See pp. 197, 220-221, and 552-553 in *Physiology* 3rd ed.)

2.   Creatine kinase is a soluble protein present in high concentrations in muscle cells. Injury or cell death and necrosis allow this enzyme and other proteins to escape and to be detected in the serum. (See pp. 296 and 327-328 in *Physiology* 3rd ed.)

3.   No, it only indicates that the normal sarcolemmal permeability barrier that retains enzymes in cells has been breached in many muscle cells. However, in a male baby born in a family with a history of Duchenne muscular dystrophy, grossly elevated levels would be a strong indication that the dystrophin gene is defective. It would be essential to determine the cause of the increased serum creatine kinase levels to avoid missing treatable diseases, such as polymyositis. (See pp. 296 and 327-328 in *Physiology* 3rd ed.)

4. The recurrent necrosis in muscle fibers balances the regenerative events. Weakness in some muscle groups for any cause leads to adaptive hypertrophic responses in synergistic muscles. The signals are unknown, although muscular activity is implicated. Clearly the regenerative processes are limited and do not balance necrosis overall. Nevertheless, variations in the stimuli for regeneration or perhaps the capacity to regenerate contribute to differential progression of the disease. (See pp. 305-307 in *Physiology* 3rd ed.)

5. This is puzzling, but two factors are implicated. One is the offsetting regenerative capacity of muscle (see answer to question 4). The other is the fact that muscle cells go through a number of developmental stages. The observation that the muscle cells of affected individuals display fetal characteristics suggests that the adult fiber phenotypes are more susceptible to the disease process or that there are developmental disturbances. (See pp. 305-306 in *Physiology* 3rd ed.)

6. The defective gene must be recessive and sex linked. Females have two X chromosomes, one from their father and one from their mother. The X chromosome from the father must contain a normal dystrophin gene (because chromosomes containing the mutation are lethal in males by adolescence). (See pp. 980-982 in *Physiology* 3rd ed.)

7. Unused motor units exhibit disuse atrophy and would exacerbate the weakness characteristic of the disease. Exercise will help preserve muscle function. (See pp. 306-307 in *Physiology* 3rd ed.)

8. Yes, in theory. In this recessive disease the mutation deprives the cells of the essential protein dystrophin. Restoration of the normal gene, if expressed, could be expected to correct or mitigate the disease. In practice, the technology to introduce a functional gene to all muscle cells does not exist.

Case 3

1. A sudden rise in cell Ca^{++} is required to initiate crossbridge cycling and contraction. This inference is supported by research showing that drugs that increase cell Ca^{++}, such as caffeine, lidocaine, and cardiac glycosides, increase the severity of the symptoms of malignant hyperthermia. Drugs that lower cell Ca^{++}, whether by preventing release from the sarcoplasmic reticulum (dantrolene) or by blocking influx through the sarcolemma (local anesthetics, Ca^{++} channel blockers), improve survival. (See pp. 292-294 in *Physiology* 3rd ed.)

2. Clinical signs include the fall in blood oxygen and pH, the rise in blood carbon dioxide, and the rise in body temperature, despite the tachycardia and increase in ventilation. (See pp. 602-604, 607-608, and 804-806 in *Physiology* 3rd ed.)

3. Skeletal muscle constitutes about 40% of the body mass, and the transition from relaxation to contraction involves a very large increase in metabolism. Therefore the contractures that result in muscle rigidity are the principal cause of increased metabolism. (See pp. 296-297 in *Physiology* 3rd ed.)

4. Both oxidative pathways (increase in carbon dioxide and decrease in oxygen) and glycolytic pathways (increase in lactate) are involved. (See p. 297 in *Physiology* 3rd ed.)

5. Normally yes, and muscle cells cease to contract (fatigue) before ATP concentrations decline. However, this is an abnormal situation where there is a failure to inactivate the tissue and reduce cell Ca^{++}. Thus glycogen depletion should be associated with reductions in creatine phosphate and ATP in fast fibers. Muscle rigidity and blood vessel compression impair blood flow, contribute to the

changes in blood gases, and limit oxidative ATP synthesis. (See pp. 298-299 and 304-305 in *Physiology* 3rd ed.)

6. Either the systems that normally reduce intracellular Ca^{++} content have failed, or increases in membrane permeability with resulting Ca^{++} diffusion into the myoplasm have overwhelmed the pumps. Increases in ATP consumption caused by crossbridge cycling and ion pumping exceed ATP production capacity. Elevated cell Na^+ and reduced cell K^+ would result, with sarcolemmal depolarization further exacerbating Ca^{++} accumulation. Cell permeability gradually increases. This causes an early loss of magnesium, phosphate, and small metabolites, followed later by the loss of soluble proteins, such as creatine kinase and myoglobin; the loss of these proteins is diagnostic of necrotic cells. (See pp. 5, 15-19, 42, and 293 in *Physiology* 3rd ed.)

7. The syndrome was triggered by agents that ordinarily inhibit Ca^{++} mobilization by blocking acetylcholine receptors at the motor end plate, thereby preventing the generation of action potentials in the sarcolemma (succinylcholine), or by a more general membrane stabilization effect (halothane). The family history suggested a genetic basis for a presumed faulty element in the excitation-contraction coupling pathways. These faulty elements include the membranes of the end plate, sarcolemma, T-tubules, and/or sarcoplasmic reticulum. (See pp. 35 and 55-57 in *Physiology* 3rd ed.)

CHAPTER 19

Case 1

1. A pressure gradient and the absence of physical barriers allow materials to move along hollow organs. (See pp. 640-642 in *Physiology* 3rd ed.)

2. Barriers to esophageal reflux include a contracted lower esophageal sphincter and a diaphragmatic pinchcock where the esophagus passes through the diaphragm. (See pp. 630-633 in *Physiology* 3rd ed.)

3. The pressures in the stomach depend on gastric smooth muscle contraction and the transmural pressure gradient from the abdominal cavity to the stomach lumen, but are always positive and typically 7 to 50 mm Hg. Because most of the esophagus is in the thoracic cavity, its mean pressure is negative and typically varies between -15 and +5 mm Hg during the respiratory cycle. Thus there is always a pressure gradient favoring reflux. This can be quite large with maximal inspiration or with contraction of the abdominal skeletal muscles that occurs in such reflexes as coughing, vomiting, and defecation. (See pp. 568, 633, and 638-639 in *Physiology* 3rd ed.)

4. The upper esophageal sphincter is a striated muscle that acts to exclude air during respiration. The proximal esophageal body contains an outer longitudinal and an inner circular striated muscle layer. There is a long transition region with two layers in which the fraction of smooth muscle increases. In humans the lower half of the esophagus contains circular and longitudinal layers of pure smooth muscle. The function of the esophageal body is to propel a bolus of food to the stomach by phasic contractions coordinated as peristalsis. The lower esophageal sphincter is smooth muscle that is distinguished from the adjacent circular body muscle more by its physiology than by its structure. The function of the lower esophageal sphincter is tonic contraction to form a barrier to prevent reflux of the gastric contents. (See pp. 630-631 in *Physiology* 3rd ed.)

5. Even though it is not attached to bone and is found in the wall of a hollow organ, the striated muscle is skeletal. The function of the body muscle of the esophagus is more like skeletal muscle than cardiac; the body muscle is normally relaxed and may be recruited voluntarily in swallowing. (See pp. 300-301 and 309 in *Physiology* 3rd ed.)

6. Both skeletal and particularly smooth muscles are very diverse. The smooth muscle of the esophagus resembles skeletal muscle with extensive innervation, generation of bursts of action potentials, and phasic contractions equivalent to a brief tetanus. However, it is not clear why primates, cats, and opossums have smooth muscle in their esophagus, whereas many other animals do not. It appears that the complex neural control mechanisms governing peristalsis in the esophagus can generate comparable mechanical responses from muscle cells that differ considerably in their contractile protein isoforms, structure, and crossbridge regulatory mechanisms. (See pp. 313-314, 318, and 321 in *Physiology* 3rd ed.)

7. Tone is dependent on Ca^{++}-stimulated crossbridge phosphorylation. Because this is a steady-state contraction, the extracellular Ca^{++} pool and the sarcolemma regulate phosphorylation. Neurotransmitters or circulating hormones are clearly not obligatory for tone, which suggests that receptor-operated channels are not of major importance. The most likely explanation is a normally low membrane potential with elevated voltage-gated Ca^{++} channel conductance. (See pp. 318-321 and 631-633 in *Physiology* 3rd ed.)

8. This must involve coordinated neural pathways and release of a neurotransmitter whose combination with a receptor produces a net reduction in cell Ca^{++}, inhibition of myosin kinase, and crossbridge dephosphorylation by myosin phosphatase. A major part of the relaxation reflects activity of vagal fibers that release VIP (vasoactive intestinal polypeptide) or NO (nitric oxide). A contributing factor is a decrease in excitatory nerve activity, such as in some cholinergic vagal fibers. (See pp. 317-319 and 633 in *Physiology* 3rd ed.)

9. Because smooth muscles can maintain tone (an isometric contraction) with as much as 300-fold lower rates of ATP consumption, the smooth muscle in the lower esophageal sphincter would be expected to be far more economical than an equivalent mass of skeletal muscle in the upper esophageal sphincter. (See pp. 319-320 in *Physiology* 3rd ed.)

10. Anything that increases the pressure gradient from the stomach to the esophagus makes reflux more likely. Gravity is one such factor. Frequent reflux with heartburn is associated with lower than normal pressures in the lower esophagus, and thus the barrier that resists the pressure gradient is too low. (See p. 633 in *Physiology* 3rd ed.)

11. Radiologic assessment is one possibility. The patient would receive a radiopaque substance, such as a barium sulfate suspension with a meal. This substance would allow detection of reflux. Another approach would be measurement of esophageal pH via a catheter, because the reflux would contain gastric acid. Direct observation is also possible with an endoscope to detect wall damage or lower esophageal sphincter patency. Also, pressure-sensing balloon catheters can be used to measure lower esophageal sphincter tone. (See p. 631 in *Physiology* 3rd ed.)

12. Several factors are involved. Ingested fats and alcohol reduce lower esophageal sphincter tone in some individuals. The acid in cola drinks (pH $\approx$ 2.3) may cause pain in an injured esophageal mucosa, as may osmotic effects. Some food and drinks (including tea and coffee) are potent stimulators of gastric acid secretion or they increase the force of gastric contractions. Although such details may not be covered in a physiology text, they are understandable in terms of activating pain receptors, increasing the pressure gradient for reflux, or decreasing the barriers to reflux. (See answers to questions 1, 3, and 10.)

Case 2

1. Narrowing of the lumen of the airways increases the resistance to air flow in and out of the lungs, and therefore increases the effort of the skeletal muscles involved in respiration. (See pp. 316 and 570-573 in *Physiology* 3rd ed.)

2. Factors that contribute to airway narrowing include the following: constriction of the smooth muscle encircling the airways, increased intrathoracic pressure that tends to compress the airways, abnormal secretion of mucus, or an inflammatory response that increases capillary permeability and thus leads to mucosal edema. (See pp. 572-573 in *Physiology* 3rd ed.)

3. Just as restricting the stem of a balloon causes turbulent air flow and the generation of sounds, airway narrowing is offset by respiratory efforts that increase the velocity of air flow and thus induce turbulence and wheezing. (See pp. 570-571 in *Physiology* 3rd ed.)

4. Airway lumen diameter is a balance between the force exerted by the airway smooth muscle against a load and of the pressure gradient between the inside and outside of the airway. On inspiration the thorax is enlarged; this reduces the pressure on the outside of the airways and causes air to flow into

the lungs. This also increases airway diameter somewhat and thus reduces the air flow resistance, turbulence, and wheezing. The pressure gradient across the wall reverses on expiration and narrows the airways. Higher flow rates result, and they cause turbulence and wheezing. (See pp. 315-316 and 570-572 in *Physiology* 3rd ed.)

5. Smooth muscle contraction reflects a balance between excitatory (constrictor) and inhibitory (dilator) agents, including neurotransmitters, circulating hormones, locally produced hormones, and drugs. These inputs may act directly on smooth muscle cells or indirectly via actions on nerves or other cells associated with the smooth muscle. Of special importance to the airways are airborne irritants or antigens, such as pollen, that act on the airway epithelia and can trigger asthmatic attacks. (See pp. 313-314, 514, and 574 in *Physiology* 3rd ed.)

6. Like the vascular system, the airways constitute an enormous network of connected tubes of various sizes. Smooth muscle is the effector cell that regulates airway diameter and thus promotes the optimum flow of air to each part of the lung. Smooth muscle constriction is also part of cough reflexes, as the increased velocity of air flow through narrowed airways helps expel mucus or irritants. (See pp. 309 and 582-584 in *Physiology* 3rd ed.)

7. Airway smooth muscle, the skeletal muscles involved in inspiration and expiration (diaphragm and intercostal muscles), and the heart and vascular smooth muscle are all involved in transporting oxygen from the lungs to the working skeletal muscles. (See p. 281 in *Physiology* 3rd ed.)

8. Fatigue occurs only in the skeletal muscles involved in inspiration and expiration, because their ATP consumption rates, attributed to crossbridge cycling, are very high because of the effort expended to overcome increased airway resistance. The muscle fatigue can prevent sufficient ventilation to meet the increased oxygen need. The resulting fall in blood oxygen and increase in carbon dioxide can lead to respiratory failure. The ATP consumption rates of smooth muscle are so much lower than those of skeletal muscle that fatigue does not occur. (See pp. 298-299, 304-305, 319-320, and 574-575 in *Physiology* 3rd ed.)

9. Not necessarily. The airway epithelium presents a barrier between the air and the smooth muscle. Hence the drug would not be effective unless it can cross the barrier. A drug that acted on the epithelial cells to cause the production and release of a relaxing agent might be more effective. In practice an asthmatic attack is usually relieved in a few minutes by drugs that are delivered in the inspired gas or intravenously and that directly or indirectly relax airway smooth muscle. (See pp. 313-316 in *Physiology* 3rd ed.)

10. Assuming that the drug crosses the alveolar-capillary membranes and reaches the vascular smooth muscle, the effect will depend on (1) the presence and density of receptors for the drug, and (2) whether receptor activation is inhibitory (as in the airway smooth muscle) or excitatory. In the latter case the pulmonary blood pressure would increase, and the systemic hypoxemia may worsen. Side effects are common, and their occurrence and nature will vary with the mode of administration of the drug. (See pp. 313-314 and 321 in *Physiology* 3rd ed.)

11. Because the resistance to air flow in expiration is greater than in inspiration (see answer to question 4), not all of the inspired air is exhaled in the initial phase of the attack. This further compromises ventilation and contributes to the dyspnea. (See pp. 572-573 in *Physiology* 3rd ed.)

12. It might block and thereby inactivate the receptor site for one of the agents that induce the contraction. Alternatively, the agent might activate a receptor that brings about relaxation by enhancing Ca^{++}

extrusion or sequestration. Some drugs block sarcolemma Ca^{++} channels to inhibit contraction. Another mechanism is to bring about hyperpolarization by stimulation of the electrogenic Na^{+}, K^{+} pump or by increasing the conductance of K^{+} channels in the sarcolemma. Drugs might also stimulate the Ca^{++} pumps to lower the myoplasmic Ca^{++}. (See pp. 320-321 in *Physiology* 3rd ed.)

Case 3

1. Contraction, proliferation, synthesis, and secretion of extracellular protein matrix. (See pp. 322-323 in *Physiology* 3rd ed.)

2. Normally myometrial smooth muscle is quiescent (relaxed), whereas cervical smooth muscle is tonically active; the latter activity serves a sphincter role. This pattern also characterizes pregnancy. Parturition is marked by rhythmic contractions of the myometrium with relaxation of cervical smooth muscle. Puberty, coitus, menses, and menopause are also associated with changes in uterine smooth muscle function. (See pp. 321 and 1020-1022 in *Physiology* 3rd ed.)

3. Men lack uterine smooth muscle, but they do have specific types of smooth muscle in the urogenital system with an embryologic origin similar to uterine smooth muscle. The urogenital system exhibits marked sexual dimorphism, but sex differences are minimal or absent in the smooth muscle of most organ systems. (See pp. 980-983 in *Physiology* 3rd ed.)

4. At the functional level, the myometrium exhibits the same spectrum of contractile activity and properties characteristic of smooth muscle in general. However, the smooth muscle of the uterus and other parts of the reproductive system is notable in its dependence on, and response to, a variety of circulating hormones (notably androgens and estrogens). (See pp. 987-988 and 997-999 in *Physiology* 3rd ed.)

5. Propagation of action potentials in smooth muscle, as in cardiac muscle, requires low–resistance junctions between the cells. In fact, gap junctions in smooth muscles are sparse during pregnancy, but they form in large numbers shortly before delivery and persist for a short time after parturition. (See p. 310 in *Physiology* 3rd ed.)

6. All of the myometrial smooth muscle cells must contract synchronously to reduce the volume of the uterus. This is achieved in most physically activated smooth muscles by electrical communication and the propagation of action potentials that originate from a pacemaker area. Contractions during pregnancy could induce miscarriages. Parturition requires forceful, coordinated activation and contraction. (See pp. 312-314 in *Physiology* 3rd ed.)

7. The formation of gap junctions involves hormonal signals. However, their precise nature remains uncertain and is highly variable among different mammalian species. A high progesterone to estrogen ratio is involved in maintaining uterine quiescence during pregnancy. (See pp. 1020-1022 in *Physiology* 3rd ed.)

8. It is the same as in all muscles: increases in the intracellular Ca^{++} concentration. (See pp. 311-312 in *Physiology* 3rd ed.)

9. In myometrial and other types of smooth muscle that generate action potentials, Ca^{++} diffusion inward through voltage-gated channels is the major cause of depolarization. Thus Ca^{++} entry from the extracellular space can contribute to activation. However, the major source of activator Ca^{++} for phasic contractions is the sarcoplasmic reticulum. (See pp. 48, 311-312, and 320-321 in *Physiology* 3rd ed.)

10. The Ca^{++} binds to calmodulin, and the resulting calmodulin-$4Ca^{++}$ complex binds to myosin kinase to activate this enzyme. Myosin kinase then phosphorylates a specific site on the crossbridges with PO_4 derived from the hydrolysis of ATP. Phosphorylated crossbridges are able to attach to the thin filaments and cycle, and thereby generate the contraction. (See pp. 286-287 and 317-319 in *Physiology* 3rd ed.)

11. After the burst of action potentials, the myoplasmic Ca^{++} concentration is reduced to low values by Ca^{++} pumps and Na^+/Ca^{++} exchangers. Ca^{++} dissociates from calmodulin, and myosin kinase reverts to its inactive form. The crossbridges are inactivated enzymatically through the removal of the PO_4 group by myosin phosphatase. (See pp. 318-321 in *Physiology* 3rd ed.)

12. First, a heartbeat is basically a twitch associated with a single action potential, whereas strong contractions of physically active single-unit smooth muscles are basically short tetani associated with a burst of action potentials. Second, the isoforms of myosin expressed in smooth muscle have intrinsically lower rates of ATP hydrolysis and crossbridge cycling. Third, covalent regulation by phosphorylation allows further reductions in cycling rates in latch, although this is of more significance for tonic smooth muscle. (See pp. 314 and 319-321 in *Physiology* 3rd ed.)

13. No. The cervical relaxation associated with myometrial contraction reflects the fact that this tonic smooth muscle is not electrically coupled to the myometrium. The normally elevated myoplasmic Ca^{++} that maintains tone and closure of the cervix is lowered as a result of reflex mechanisms that trigger relaxation. (See p. 320 in *Physiology* 3rd ed.)

14. All the elements of the myometrium, including smooth muscle, blood vessels, other cell types, and the extracellular matrix, increase. Increases in smooth muscle mass result from proliferation (hyperplasia) and growth in cell size (hypertrophy). Smooth muscle also contributes to the extracellular matrix through synthesis and secretion of proteins, such as collagen. (See pp. 322-323 in *Physiology* 3rd ed.)

15. These are poorly understood, diverse, and quite variable among mammals. The gonadal steroids clearly are important. (See pp. 1012 and 1016-1019 in *Physiology* 3rd ed.)

Case 4

1. Two principal factors make this possible. (1) The load on the smooth muscle is the tangential wall stress, and this falls as the radius decreases. (2) The vascular wall is essentially incompressible; hence, constriction leads to increased wall thickness and decreased lumen diameter. (See p. 316 in *Physiology* 3rd ed.)

2. No. Blood flow to the digits is important in temperature regulation and the cutaneous fraction of the total hand blood flow is relatively high. The vessels constrict rhythmically in the digits and the frequency decreases as the environment warms. The vascular system will shift blood flow to tissues with increased needs, such as working muscle. For example, blood flow to the leg muscles is increased during bicycle exercise but blood flow to the fingers is reduced. (See pp. 517-518 in *Physiology* 3rd ed.)

3. Although core temperature is maintained during cold exposure, the temperature of the extremities will fall below 37° C. Enzymatic activity is highly temperature dependent; therefore all aspects of muscle function will be depressed. (See p. 518 in *Physiology* 3rd ed.)

4. Because crossbridge regulation by phosphorylation depends on the enzymes myosin kinase and myosin phosphatase, the events that link activation and contraction are potentially more temperature dependent in smooth muscle. Some smooth muscles (piloerector and cutaneous vascular smooth muscle) may be exposed to reduced temperatures because of their superficial location. (See pp. 318-319 in *Physiology* 3rd ed.)

5. Lower temperatures would reduce the rates of ATP synthesis, but this would be offset by reduced rates of ATP consumption. Rigor mortis does not occur physiologically, and fatigue processes inhibit muscle contraction before ATP levels are reduced. Furthermore, the extraordinary high economy of force maintenance by vascular smooth muscle makes it comparatively insensitive to metabolic limitations. (See pp. 304-305 and 319-320 in *Physiology* 3rd ed.)

6. The specific answer is uncertain, although glycolysis can provide ATP during a period of anoxia. However, sufficient circulation must be maintained to prevent cell death over longer periods. Intermittent or collateral circulation must meet the minimum requirements of the cooled tissues for survival. (See 296-297 in *Physiology* 3rd ed.)

7. Apart from skin pigments the color is mainly a function of the amount of blood in the cutaneous venous plexus. Coloration from red to blue is attributable to the degree of saturation of hemoglobin by oxygen in the red blood cells. (See p. 519 in *Physiology* 3rd ed.)

8. A spasm usually refers to a sudden, violent, involuntary and painful contraction of a muscle. However, a vasospasm is neither violent nor painful (although the downstream loss of flow may induce intense pain, as in a coronary vasospasm). In the absence of a skeleton, the muscle shortens to a length that occludes the vessel while it reduces the forces generated. (See p. 316 in *Physiology* 3rd ed.)

9. Interruption of flow is followed by reactive hyperemia: an elevation of flow above preocclusion levels, caused by accumulated vasodilator metabolites that relax vascular smooth muscle. Many vasodilators elevate cyclic nucleotide levels in smooth muscle cells. (See pp. 322 and 484 in *Physiology* 3rd ed.)

10. As part of the body's thermoregulation mechanism, warming normally induces vasodilation, whereas cooling induces vasoconstriction. However, prolonged, severe cold leads to a secondary vasodilation. (See p. 518 in *Physiology* 3rd ed.)

11. Peripheral temperature receptors and the sympathetic nervous system mediate the response of cutaneous blood vessels to temperature. Also, cooled blood that reaches the anterior hypothalamus will produce reflex cutaneous vasoconstriction. Constriction of blood vessels is typically caused by increases in sympathetic nerve activity, whereas reduced sympathetic nerve activity is associated with vasodilation. The arteriovenous anastomoses prominent in the fingers and toes are entirely under neural control. (See pp. 517-518 in *Physiology* 3rd ed.)

12. Because a precipitating cause of the three conditions is digital, cerebral, and coronary vasospasm, respectively, this "coincidence" suggests that there may be some generalized vascular abnormality. However, the digital vasculature has strong neural control, the coronary vessels—less so, and the cerebral vessels—negligible neural regulation. Hence a common factor is not obvious. (See pp. 529-530 in *Physiology* 3rd ed.)

13. An acute vasodilation would be expected, because these vessels have an extensive sympathetic innervation and lack parasympathetic vasodilator fibers. Unlike skeletal muscle, smooth muscle can survive and maintain function after denervation. (See pp. 322 and 518 in *Physiology* 3rd ed.)

14. Unlike denervated skeletal muscle, in which the motor nerve bodies remain intact and can grow from the severed axon and reinnervate cells, the cell bodies of fibers in the sympathetic ganglia would be destroyed by denervation procedures. The return of tone is probably caused by denervation hypersensitivity or supersensitivity to circulating catecholamines. These changes in sensitivity result from an increase in the number of receptors on the smooth muscle cells. Supersensitivity also occurs in denervated skeletal muscle cells, as receptors for acetylcholine are no longer limited to the motor end plate. (See pp. 306, 322, and 518 in *Physiology* 3rd ed.)

15. Yes. Tone is the balance between mechanisms that tend to increase myoplasmic Ca^{++} and those that tend to reduce it. A loss of the latter would lead to vasospasm. Although cutaneous blood vessels do not have vasodilator nerves, they relax in response to circulating or locally produced metabolites or other vasodilators. (See pp. 320-322 in *Physiology* 3rd ed.)

CHAPTER 20

1. A complete blood count including hematocrit (the proportionate volume of red blood cells in a given volume of blood, measured after blood is centrifuged in a standardized way), hemoglobin levels, red and white blood cell counts, platelet count, and examination of a stained blood smear. (See pp. 329-330 in *Physiology* 3rd ed.)

2. The red blood cell count is only slightly below normal, but the hematocrit and the concentration of hemoglobin are sharply reduced. These findings are typical of hypochromic microcytic anemia, that is, anemia in which the number of red blood cells is reduced, and, on average, the hemoglobin content of individual red blood cells is also reduced. (See p. 330 in *Physiology* 3rd ed.)

3. (a) Examination of a stained blood smear. This would confirm the diagnosis, because the red blood cells would be excessively pale, and their size and shape, normally monotonous, may vary widely. (b) Measurement of the concentrations of serum iron and of its carrier protein, transferrin (iron-binding globulin). In this case, serum iron was drastically reduced, and the concentration of iron-binding globulin was elevated. These findings help to distinguish iron deficiency anemia from certain other anemias, such as those caused by hereditary disorders of hemoglobin synthesis and structure. (c) Measurement of serum ferritin, which is diminished in patients with low iron stores even before the falling hematocrit. (d) Examination of bone marrow by using stains that detect iron. In this patient, no iron could be detected, as if the loss of iron were not acute but of long standing. (See pp. 329-330 in *Physiology* 3rd ed.)

4. Ferrous sulfate is readily absorbed from the lumen of the duodenum. The iron, attached to plasma transferrin, is carried to erythrocyte precursors in marrow, where it is internalized, separated from the carrier protein, and used for synthesis of heme. (See pp. 329-330 in *Physiology* 3rd ed.)

5. If bleeding continues, this may be difficult to do. If appropriate therapy of peptic ulcer is successful, administration of iron may be followed within days by a rise in the number of reticulocytes in peripheral blood as newly formed erythrocytes enter the blood stream. Within about 2 weeks the red blood cell count, hemoglobin levels, and hematocrit all rise. (See pp. 329-330 in *Physiology* 3rd ed.)

CHAPTER 21

1. Platelets accumulate at the site of vascular endothelial damage, adhere to the site of injury, and clump together to form a plug that can seal small injuries. Platelets also promote clotting by furnishing phospholipids (needed for clotting) and receptors (for plasma-clotting factors that potentiate the clotting process). (See pp. 353-356 in *Physiology* 3rd ed.)

   In the second test, blood is drawn into a solution of sodium citrate, the plasma is separated by centrifugation, tissue thromboplastin is added to the plasma, and a solution of calcium chloride is added to the mixture. The interval until the mixture clots is designated as the *prothrombin time*, and the normal value is usually 12 to 14 seconds. This patient's prothrombin time was 12.5 seconds.

2. Sodium citrate forms a soluble complex with plasma calcium ions, and it inhibits clotting. Addition of calcium chloride after addition of tissue thromboplastin restores these necessary ions and allows clotting to proceed. The prothrombin time is a measure of the extrinsic pathway of thrombin formation; it is called extrinsic because tissue thromboplastin is not a normal constituent of plasma. (See pp. 347-348 in *Physiology* 3rd ed.)

3. (a) Deficiency of any plasma constituents of the extrinsic pathway, except calcium ions (which are added from a bottle), and of fibrin-stabilizing factor (factor XIII), which acts to form covalent bonds between adjacent fibrin monomers. (b) The presence of an abnormal inhibitor of thrombin formation, for example, therapeutically administered heparin. (c) The presence of an extrinsic pathway clotting factor that is structurally abnormal; hence a clot cannot form within a normal time. The most common such defect is the presence of a species of fibrinogen that has an amino acid substitution that results in delayed clotting. (See pp. 341-348 in *Physiology* 3rd ed.)

   In the third test, blood is drawn into a solution of sodium citrate (as for the prothrombin time), the plasma is separated, and the clotting time is measured after sequential additions to the plasma of a suspension of phospholipids and a solution of calcium chloride. The term *partial thromboplastin* is derived from the fact that tissue thromboplastin is a complex of phospholipids and protein. In contrast to the prothrombin time, here only the phospholipid moiety of tissue thromboplastin is added to plasma. The normal partial thromboplastin time, as usually measured, varies from about 25 to 32 seconds. In this patient the partial thromboplastin time was 52 seconds.

4. Because the prothrombin time is normal, one must assume that the patient's clotting abnormality lies within the early steps of the intrinsic pathway of thrombin formation before the participation of Stuart factor (factor X), proaccelerin (factor V), prothrombin (factor II), and fibrin-stabilizing factor (factor XIII or fibrinogen). (See pp. 344-347 in *Physiology* 3rd ed.)

5. Hageman factor (factor XII), plasma prekallikrein, high-molecular-weight kininogen, plasma thromboplastin antecedent (PTA, factor XI), antihemophilic factor (factor VIII), and Christmas factor (factor IX). (See pp. 344-345 in *Physiology* 3rd ed.)

6. The disorder appears to be caused by a defect on the X chromosome. Testing of the patient's relatives may be necessary to confirm this presumption. (See p. 346 in *Physiology* 3rd ed.)

7. Again, deficiency of a clotting factor, the presence of an inhibitor of the clotting process (e.g., heparin), or the presence of a structurally abnormal protein that does not support normal clotting. (See pp. 346-347 in *Physiology* 3rd ed.)

8. Hereditary deficiencies of Hageman factor (factor XII), plasma prekallikrein, and high-molecular-weight kininogen are not accompanied by a bleeding tendency. Also, deficiency of plasma thromoplastin antecedent (PTA, factor XI) either causes no symptoms or is accompanied by only mild evidence of a bleeding tendency. Anyway, all these deficiencies are inherited in an autosomal recessive manner; that is, the abnormal gene is located on a chromosome other than the X chromosome, and it must be inherited from both parents. (See pp. 344-347 in *Physiology* 3rd ed.)

9. A deficiency of either antihemophilic factor (factor VIII) or Christmas factor (factor IX) would explain the patient's symptoms. To test this, the patient's plasma is mixed with that of patients with either classic hemophilia (factor VIII deficiency) or Christmas disease (factor IX deficiency). Determination of the partial thromboplastin time of the mixture will indicate which factor the patient lacks. In the present case, the partial thromboplastin time of the mixture of the patient's plasma with the plasma deficient in Christmas factor (factor IX) shortened the partial thromboplastin time to 28 seconds. This indicates that the patient was deficient in factor VIII, which was furnished by the plasma deficient in factor IX. (See pp. 344-348 in *Physiology* 3rd ed.)

   The fourth test, the bleeding time, is the time it takes for bleeding to stop after a small, deliberately incised wound; several different techniques have been described. Paradoxically, the bleeding time is usually normal in defects of blood coagulation. It was normal in the present instance.

10. The bleeding time measures hemostasis at the site of a minor injury to the blood vessel wall. It is not surprising, then, to learn that the bleeding time is abnormally long if too few platelets are present in the circulating blood (thrombocytopenia) or if the circulating platelets are abnormal (thrombocytopathia). The bleeding time is not expected to be long when the number of circulating platelets is greatly increased (thrombocytosis or thrombocythemia); the mechanism is not clear.

   In the present case, we know that the patient's plasma is deficient in factor VIII (antihemophilic factor).

11. In patients with classic hemophilia, the bleeding time is normal. In those with von Willebrand's disease, the bleeding time is long because the patient's plasma is deficient in von Willebrand factor, which is needed to promote adhesion of platelets to the edges of the vascular injury created by the deliberately incised wound. Von Willebrand's disease can be further distinguished from hemophilia, because its mode of inheritance is autosomal dominant and not X chromosome linked. (See p. 346 in *Physiology* 3rd ed.)

12. Because the patient's mother is clearly a carrier of classic hemophilia, his sister has an even chance of inheriting the normal gene supporting synthesis of factor VIII or the abnormal gene. (See p. 346 in *Physiology* 3rd ed.)

CHAPTER 22

1. The wound in the left arm with the pulsatile bleeding is more serious because it is indicative of a severed artery. Blood loss from the artery is rapid because of the higher pressure, compared with blood loss from the neck vein where the pressure is much lower. (See pp. 361-362 in *Physiology* 3rd ed.)

2. The pulsations are caused by the intermittent ejection of blood by the left ventricle. The venous bleeding is nonpulsatile because the pulsations have been damped out in the microcirculation (arterioles and capillaries). (See pp. 361-362 in *Physiology* 3rd ed.)

3. Blood flow velocity would be fastest in the arteries that have the smallest total cross-sectional area, and slowest in the capillaries that have the largest total cross-sectional area. (See pp. 361-362 in *Physiology* 3rd ed.)

4. Blood pressure decreases along the vascular tree from aorta to vena cava. (If there were not a pressure gradient from the arterial to the venous side of the circulation, there could not be flow of blood in this direction). (See pp. 361-362 in *Physiology* 3rd ed.)

5. The greatest pressure drop occurs across the arterioles, sometimes called the "stopcocks" of the circulation. Resistance to blood flow is greatest in the arterioles. (See pp. 361-362 in *Physiology* 3rd ed.)

6. Most of the blood is located in the veins of the circulatory system, mainly in the large and medium-sized veins. (See pp. 361-362 in *Physiology* 3rd ed.)

CHAPTER 23

1. As the K^+ concentration rises in the interstitial fluid of the ischemic zone, the ratio of the intracellular K^+ concentration ($[K^+]_i$) to the extracellular K^+ concentration ($[K^+]_o$) would decrease. The myocardial cell membranes at rest (phase 4) are much more permeable to K^+ than to any other relevant ion. Hence, the resting membrane potential is very close to that estimated by the Nernst equation for K^+. As the $[K^+]_i/K[^+]_o$ ratio diminishes, the resting membrane potential becomes less negative, as predicted by the Nernst equation. (See p. 366 in *Physiology* 3rd ed.)

2. The fast Na^+ channels in the myocardial cell membranes are voltage sensitive. As the resting membrane potential of myocardial cells becomes progressively less negative (i.e., partially depolarized), more and more of the fast Na^+ channels in those cells become inactivated because of their voltage dependency. Hence, when the wave of excitation reaches the partially depolarized cells, a diminished number of fast Na^+ channels are available to be activated. The upstroke of the action potential in myocardial cells is mediated by the influx of Na^+ through the fast Na^+ channels. In the myocardial cells in the ischemic zone of the heart, fewer Na^+ channels are available for activation than in the myocardial cells in the normal regions of the heart. Therefore, in the ischemic cells, the upstroke of the action potential is less steep than normal, and the amplitude of the action potential is diminished. The velocity of impulse propagation varies directly with the amplitude and with the slope of the upstroke of the action potential. Hence, propagation is abnormally slow in the ischemic zone. (See p. 375 in *Physiology* 3rd ed.)

3. Localized regions of slow conduction may lead to unidirectional block, which is one prerequisite for reentry. The unidirectional block is often a temporal phenomenon; that is, part of a given wave of excitation may approach a given site in the heart from one direction. If it travels through normal tissue, it may arrive early at the given site, at a time when the site is still refractory from a preceding depolarization. However, if another part of the same wave of excitation arrives at the same site from a different direction, but reaches the site later because of a local conduction delay, the given site may then have recovered from its refractory period and be excitable. Hence, the impulse will now be conducted through the given site, but in a different direction. Such "unidirectional block" can lead to premature depolarizations or paroxysmal tachycardias, by virtue of reentrant conduction. (See pp. 385 and 391-394 in *Physiology* 3rd ed.)

4. In resting myocardial cells, the cell membrane is much more permeable to K^+ than to any other relevant ion, but it is virtually impermeable to Na^+. Hence, inactivation of the fast Na^+ channels will have no detectable effect on the resting membrane potential. (See p. 367 in *Physiology* 3rd ed.)

5. As more and more fast Na^+ channels are inactivated by the antiarrhythmic drug, the action potential upstroke would become less steep, and the propagation velocity would diminish, as explained in answer 2 above. (See also pp. 367 and 375 in *Physiology* 3rd ed.)

6. A drug that affects only fast Na^+ channels would have a negligible effect on action potentials of SA node cells or of conduction fibers in the N region of the AV node, because these cardiac cells are "slow response" fibers. The upstrokes of their action potentials depend mainly on influx of Ca^{++} through Ca^{++} channels, rather than on influx of Na^+, as in myocardial cells. Also, the slow diastolic depolarization in the SA node cells is mediated by changes in the conductance of K^+, Ca^{++}, and Na^+. Furthermore, the channels that conduct the Na^+ during the slow diastolic depolarization are the so-called i_f current channels, not the fast Na^+ current channels. (See pp. 374 and 380 in *Physiology* 3rd ed.)

7. The firing rate of the SA node cells would diminish as a consequence of the increased vagal activity. The acetylcholine (ACh) released from the vagus nerve endings activates the ACh-regulated K^+ channels and decreases the conductance of the i_f channels. The increased K^+ conductance tends to hyperpolarize the automatic cell membranes, and therefore the transmembrane potential at the beginning of slow diastolic depolarization is more negative than it is in the absence of vagal activity. This would tend to increase the cardiac cycle length (i.e., decrease heart rate). Also, the vagally induced diminution of the conductance of the i_f channels would reduce the influx of Na^+ into the cell, and would thereby decrease the slope of slow diastolic depolarization. This also would tend to decrease heart rate. (See pp. 378-381 in *Physiology* 3rd ed.)

8. Increased vagal activity tends to retard AV conduction; that is, the time from the beginning of atrial depolarization to the beginning of ventricular depolarization may be prolonged. Intense vagal activity may even prevent the cardiac impulse from being propagated from the atria to the ventricles. The ACh released from the vagus nerve endings in the AV node activates the ACh-regulated K^+ channels and thereby hyperpolarizes the conducting fibers in the AV node. The neurally released ACh also tends to decrease the Ca^{++} current through the Ca^{++} channels in the cell membranes of the conducting fibers (which are slow-response fibers). The effects of the ACh on the K^+ and Ca^{++} currents tend to impede AV conduction.

   These direct inhibitory effects of neurally released ACh on AV conduction are moderated by the indirect dromotropic effect that vagal activity exerts by decreasing heart rate. AV conduction tends to vary inversely with heart rate; that is, the greater the frequency at which the atrial impulses reach the AV node, the slower will those impulses be conducted through the AV junction, and vice versa. Increased vagal activity will diminish the heart rate. This reduced heart rate will tend to facilitate AV conduction, and will thereby attenuate the inhibitory effect that neurally released ACh will exert directly on the AV node conducting fiber. (See pp. 382-383 in *Physiology* 3rd ed.)

9. When conduction in the AV node or bundle of His is blocked, the atrial and ventricular rhythms are "dissociated." The atrial rhythm will be set by the SA node, and the atrial rate will usually be between 60 and 90 beats/min. The ventricular rhythm will be set by specialized conduction (Purkinje) fibers, which would discharge at rates of about 30 to 45 beats/min. (See pp. 380 and 391 in *Physiology* 3rd ed.)

10. When automatic cells, such as Purkinje fibers, are driven at a rate greater than their normal firing frequency, excessive amounts of Na^+ enter the cells during each depolarization. Hence, the pump (Na^+,K^+-ATPase) operates at an accelerated rate to extrude the excess intracellular Na^+. The Na^+ pump is an electrogenic pump, in that it ejects 3 Na^+ for every 2 K^+ that it pulls in. This disparity in cation exchange tends to hyperpolarize the cell. When the overdrive ceases (i.e., when the artificial pacemaker stops firing), the activity of the Na^+ pump returns gradually toward normal, and hence the hyperpolarization is dissipated rather slowly. This retards the rate at which the Purkinje fibers in the ventricles regain their normal firing frequency. This delay in the return to normal activity by a period of high-frequency stimulation is called *overdrive suppression*. (See p. 381 in *Physiology* 3rd ed.)

CHAPTER 24

1. Cardiac output would be slow as a result of a decreased stroke volume. The reason for the reduced stroke volume is a weakened myocardium, resulting from ischemic damage from an inadequate coronary blood supply (severe narrowing of the coronary arteries). The curve of developed pressure versus diastolic filling pressure (Starling curve) would be shifted to the right and would be flatter than the normal curve. (See pp. 397 and 503 in *Physiology* 3rd ed.)

2. The neck vein distension and the liver enlargement indicate that the right ventricle is unable to pump out the large volume of blood present on the venous side of the circulation. This large volume of venous blood is caused by a shift of blood from the arterial to the venous side secondary to the reduced cardiac output and by an increase in total blood volume, resulting from the reduced cardiac output → decreased renal blood flow → increased aldosterone secretion → sodium retention → water retention. This back pressure in the venous system leads to swelling of the liver. (See pp. 398, 489, and 503 in *Physiology* 3rd ed.)

3. The efficiency of the heart is reduced in this patient with heart failure. The heart is greatly dilated, and more energy is required to eject the same volume of blood per beat than is required in the normal heart. This can be explained by the Laplace equation:

$$\sigma = P \times r / w$$

where σ (stress) is the force per unit area of cross-section of the ventricular wall, P is the pressure in the left ventricle, r is the radius of the left ventricle, and w is the thickness of the left ventricular wall. In this patient, the left ventricle is greatly dilated. Therefore the r value is large and results in an increase in σ, that is, in the force that each unit area of myocardial fibers must generate. P and w are within normal limits. (See pp. 398 and 516 in *Physiology* 3rd ed.)

4. The ejection fraction, the fraction of the end-diastolic volume ejected with each beat (stroke volume) is low, and the residual volume (amount of blood remaining in the ventricle at the end of ejection) is high. When the heart is dilated and its contractility is reduced, as in this patient with heart failure, the weak ventricular contractions eject less than the normal stroke volume. This, coupled with a large volume of blood in the ventricle during diastole and systole, greatly decreases the ejection fraction. (See pp. 405 and 410 in *Physiology* 3rd ed.)

5. Digitalis was given to increase the contractility of the heart; that is, at a constant preload and afterload, the force of contraction is enhanced. By poisoning the Na^+, K^+-ATPase, less Na^+ is pumped out of the myocardial cells. As a result, the Na^+-Ca^{++} exchange is reversed and less Ca^{++} leaves the myocytes. The greater intracellular Ca^{++} increases the cardiac contractile force. (See p. 402 in *Physiology* 3rd ed.)

6. A calcium channel antagonist would not be useful, because a greater intracellular calcium is needed to enhance myocardial contractility in this patient. However, the calcium antagonist could reduce afterload by relaxing the vascular smooth muscles of the arterioles. (See p. 402 in *Physiology* 3rd ed.)

7. Norepinephrine would increase myocardial contractility, which would be beneficial. However, it also increases heart rate and peripheral resistance, which would be deleterious. A catecholamine that is sometimes used in heart failure is dobutamine, which has less effect on heart rate and peripheral

resistance. Catecholamines act mainly by increasing intracellular calcium. (See p. 402 in *Physiology* 3rd ed.)

8. A phlebotomy would relieve the venous distension and ease the large preload on the heart. However, it is only indicated when there is acute, life-threatening pulmonary edema, and even then, tourniquets on the extremities are more commonly used. The best way to ease the preload burden on the heart is by the use of diuretics. A transfusion would be contraindicated, because it would increase the already high preload. (See pp. 398 and 503 in *Physiology* 3rd ed.)

9. The diastolic gallop rhythm indicates severe heart disease and is caused by vibrations of the ventricle walls. The vibrations are elicited by abrupt cessation of ventricular distension and the deceleration of the entering blood when the ventricle is stretched to the point that it becomes stiff. (See p. 410 in *Physiology* 3rd ed.)

10. Contractility is reduced, and the cardiac fibers are stretched beyond their optimal length so that the actin and myosin filaments do not have sufficient overlap for maximal crossbridge activity. dP/dt serves as an index of contractility. It is the maximal rate of pressure development during ventricular systole. (See pp. 404 and 405 in *Physiology* 3rd ed.)

11. Atrial contraction is relatively unimportant in ventricular filling in this patient because of the high venous pressure and the large residual volume of blood in the ventricles. The atrial contribution to ventricular filling is more important in normal hearts, especially at fast heart rates. (See p. 412 in *Physiology* 3rd ed.)

12. Peripheral resistance is increased. With a low cardiac output, arterial pressure would decrease and activate the baroreceptor reflex, which enhances peripheral resistance and thereby maintains blood pressure. (See pp. 459 and 486 in *Physiology* 3rd ed.)

13. Increased heart rate is a compensatory mechanism that is mediated by the baroreceptor reflex. The increased heart rate and the increased peripheral resistance are both elicited by the reduced blood pressure, which is caused by the decrease in cardiac output. (See p. 420 in *Physiology* 3rd ed.)

14. Reducing preload would take some of the stress off the dilated ventricles and allow the heart to move back to a more optimal functioning position on the Starling curve (from descending limb to ascending limb). Of course, if the cardiac muscle fibers were optimally stretched by the large volume of blood in diastole, then a decrease in preload would reduce cardiac output. An increase in preload would push the heart further to the right on the Starling curve (descending limb) and decrease its pumping action. (See p. 403 in *Physiology* 3rd ed.)

15. Increasing afterload would place an additional burden on the left ventricle, and cardiac output would decrease. Decreasing the afterload with the use of vasodilators (decrease peripheral resistance) can be helpful in the treatment of patients with heart failure. (See p. 403 in *Physiology* 3rd ed.)

16. The arteriovenous oxygen difference would be expected to be greater than normal because the venous blood oxygen content would be low. With a low cardiac output and hence a low blood flow through the peripheral tissues, more oxygen is extracted from the blood in the capillaries. Even with greater oxygen extraction the oxygen supply is less than optimal for the muscles. The reduced supply of oxygen can account in part for the feeling of weakness and fatigue. (See p. 533 in *Physiology* 3rd ed.)

17. Both force of contraction and velocity of contraction are decreased in this patient's heart as a result of the "heart failure" caused by inadequate blood supply to the myocardial fibers over a period of many years. (See pp. 403 and 404 in *Physiology* 3rd ed.)

18. Yes, valve function is apparently normal. However, with severe dilation of the ventricles, the valve rings can be overstretched and produce valve insufficiency, causing cardiac murmurs. (See p. 407 in *Physiology* 3rd ed.)

19. The heart sounds are probably normal, although they may be slightly diminished because of the relatively weak cardiac contractions. (See p. 409 in *Physiology* 3rd ed.)

20. Because of prolonged inadequate blood supply, the myocardial fibers contract less effectively. In addition, an increase in blood volume caused by salt and water retention by the kidneys, in response to a low cardiac output, contributes to the dilation of the heart. (See pp. 397 and 503 in *Physiology* 3rd ed.)

21. Although the heart is made up of millions of individual muscle fibers, the ventricular fibers contract together as do the atrial fibers because the heart functions as a syncytium. That is, the electrical impulse spreads rapidly from cell to cell through very low-resistance pathways called gap junctions. (See p. 398 in *Physiology* 3rd ed.)

22. The Fick principle could be used to measure cardiac output. This method would require measurements of oxygen consumption and oxygen content of mixed venous (pulmonary artery) blood and of arterial blood. A simpler and more widely used method is thermodilution. (See pp. 412-415 in *Physiology* 3rd ed.)

23. The patient is short of breath because (1) excess fluid in the lung interstitium makes the lungs stiff, which in turn requires a greater effort to expand them; and (2) fluid in the alveoli of the lung bases (rales and x-ray density) interferes with gas exchange, especially the diffusion of oxygen from alveoli to pulmonary capillaries. (See pp. 474 and 581 in *Physiology* 3rd ed.)

24. The leg edema is caused by the increased hydrostatic pressure in the capillaries and venules in the legs. The large blood volume and high venous pressure cause the hydrostatic pressure to exceed the oncotic pressure, particularly in the dependent parts of the body. This results in movement of fluid from the vascular compartment to the interstitial compartment. When the patient is bedridden, the hydrostatic pressure is greatest over the sacral region (most dependent part of the body), and sacral edema occurs. (See p. 474 in *Physiology* 3rd ed.)

25. A diuretic was given to increase sodium excretion in the urine. The diuretic reduces the reabsorption of sodium in the renal tubules and thereby increases the loss of sodium and accompanying water. (See p. 782 in *Physiology* 3rd ed.)

26. The intake of salt would be restricted to prevent edema (peripheral and pulmonary) and ascites. (See p. 770 in *Physiology* 3rd ed.)

CHAPTER 25

1. Action potentials recorded from efferent nerve fibers to the heart in experimental animals indicate that sympathetic activity increases and vagal activity decreases during inspiration. The opposite changes take place during expiration. (See p. 422 in *Physiology* 3rd ed.)

2. The changes in activity in both divisions of the autonomic nervous system would tend to contribute to the respiratory sinus arrhythmia (i.e., to the observed alterations in heart rate throughout the respiratory cycle). However, when atropine (which blocks the cardiac effects of the vagal activity) is given, the respiratory sinus arrhythmia usually disappears entirely. However, when propranolol (which blocks the cardiac effects of the sympathetic activity) is given, the respiratory sinus arrhythmia is scarcely affected.

   The vagal influence usually predominates over the sympathetic influence as a mediator of respiratory sinus arrhythmia for several reasons. First, in normal resting individuals, vagal activity is usually substantial, whereas sympathetic activity is usually minimal. Second, this disparity in activity is usually exaggerated in people who exercise regularly. Third, and probably most important, the time courses of the vagal and sympathetic effects on the heart are entirely different. The vagal effects produce their responses very quickly (relative to the duration of a respiratory cycle), and the vagal responses also decay very quickly after vagal activity ceases. Conversely, the onset and decay of the cardiac responses to sympathetic activity are much more sluggish. Periodic changes in sympathetic activity associated with the respiratory cycle cannot produce appreciable changes in cardiac function within the usual time course of a respiratory cycle, because the cardiac changes develop so slowly at the beginning of any brief period of sympathetic activity and the cardiac changes also decay very slowly after the sympathetic activity ceases. (See p. 422 in *Physiology* 3rd ed.)

3. The failure of propranolol to induce any substantial change in mean heart rate or in the respiratory fluctuations in heart rate does not necessarily signify that the activity in the cardiac sympathetic nerves was negligible. The slow heart rate (55 beats/min) and the prominent respiratory sinus arrhythmia suggest that the vagal tone in this patient was considerable. Under such conditions, the vagal influence on heart rate would predominate, even if sympathetic activity also was substantial. The summation of sympathetic and vagal effects on heart rate is highly nonlinear. One of the principal mechanisms responsible for the vagal predominance is that the acetylcholine released from vagal nerve endings acts to inhibit the release of norepinephrine from neighboring sympathetic nerve endings. Thus even if sympathetic neural activity were substantial, the sympathetic nerve endings might not release much norepinephrine if the tissue concentration of acetylcholine were appreciable in the region of the sympathetic nerve terminals. Under such conditions, propranolol would probably have little influence on heart rate. (See pp. 417-418 in *Physiology* 3rd ed.)

4. When a ventricular depolarization is very premature (as in R′ in Fig. 25-1), the time for ventricular filling is severely limited, the sarcomeres will not be stretched optimally, and therefore the contractions will be weak (Frank-Starling mechanism). Furthermore, premature depolarization affects the intracellular Ca^{++} distribution and hence the strength of contraction. During each heartbeat, the Ca^{++} that dissociates from the contractile proteins is rapidly taken up by the sarcoplasmic reticulum (SR) during relaxation. However, several hundred milliseconds must elapse before that Ca^{++} is fully available to be released again by the SR. Hence, very premature contractions are associated with a meager release of Ca^{++} from the SR, and therefore the premature contraction is feeble. In the patient whose tracings are shown in Fig. 25-1, the premature contraction evidently did not generate a sufficiently high intraventricular pressure to force open the aortic valves and to eject blood into the aorta. Therefore the premature contraction had no evident effect on the aortic pressure tracing.

5. The same factors operate, but in the opposite direction, to explain the large pulse pressure for the contraction after the premature beat (Fig. 25-1). The long pause (compensatory pause) after the premature beat allowed a prolonged filling time for the ventricles, and therefore the increased sarcomere stretch augmented the cardiac contraction (Frank-Starling mechanism). Furthermore, the compensatory pause also allowed more than sufficient time for the sarcoplasmic reticulum to release the Ca^{++} that had been taken up during both the premature beat and the beat that preceded it. Therefore the contraction that followed the premature beat could eject a supernormal stroke volume and thereby produce the large arterial pulse pressure. (See pp. 392, 429-431, and 460 in *Physiology* 3rd ed.)

6. The baroreceptor reflex is probably the principal mechanism responsible for the alternating P-P intervals (Fig. 25-2) that are often observed in patients with 2:1 AV block. This distinctive rhythm, which is referred to as ventriculophasic sinus arrhythmia, is characterized by cyclic fluctuations in arterial blood pressure (P_a) associated with the alternating presence and absence of a ventricular contraction during consecutive P-P intervals. During the cardiac cycles in which the ventricles contract and eject blood, P_a rises from its diastolic value to its systolic value, and then begins to fall again. During such a cycle, the arterial baroreceptors are stimulated by the rise in P_a, and after a brief delay, they increase cardiac vagal activity and decrease cardiac sympathetic activity. During the alternate cycles, the ventricles fail to contract, and therefore P_a falls below the level attained at the end of the preceding cardiac cycle. Hence, vagal activity progressively diminishes and sympathetic activity rises.

    Usually the reflex delay initiated by the systolic rise in P_a is sufficiently long that it does not prolong the concurrent cardiac cycle. Instead, the ventricular contraction usually causes the subsequent P-P interval (one that does not include an R wave) to be prolonged. Occasionally, however, the temporal relation between the reflex delay and the cardiac cycle length is such that those P-P intervals that do contain the R waves are the intervals that are prolonged, and the P-P intervals that do not include an R wave are abridged. (See pp. 417-420 in *Physiology* 3rd ed.)

7. Although the cyclic alternation in P_a does alter both vagal and sympathetic neural activity in each cardiac cycle, the alternating changes in P-P interval can usually be abolished completely by atropine, but propranolol will have little influence. The main reason for this is that vagally mediated cardiac responses can be initiated and terminated rapidly, within the time constraints of an ordinary cardiac cycle, whereas sympathetically mediated responses are much more sluggish and cannot induce appreciable changes beat by beat. (See pp. 418-420 in *Physiology* 3rd ed.)

CHAPTER 26

1. A catheter with an end-hole that faces upstream records the *total pressure* in a flowing stream; that is, it records the sum of a *dynamic pressure* (P_{dy}) component and a *static pressure* (P_{st}) component. However, a side-hole catheter will record only P_{st}. Hence, the difference (25 mm Hg) in the pressures recorded by the two types of catheters will equal the dynamic pressure component, P_{dy}. This pressure component reflects the influence of the kinetic energy of the moving fluid. P_{dy} equals $\rho v^2/2$ (or 33,250 dynes/cm^2), where ρ is the density of the blood (about 1.06), and v is the velocity of the flowing blood. Hence the peak velocity of the blood flowing through the aortic valve orifice must have been about 258 cm/sec. (See pp. 439-440 in *Physiology* 3rd ed.)

2. Generally, in vascular beds, including the coronary vascular bed, the resistance per unit length is normally very small in the major distributing arteries, but it is substantial in the small "resistance" vessels. Hence in a normal left circumflex coronary artery, the pressure drop per cm length along the vessel is negligible. Let us assume that the normal drop in pressure per unit length is 0.1 mm Hg per cm of vessel length at the normal rate of blood flow through the vessel. Because resistance (R) equals pressure drop (ΔP) divided by flow (Q), the pressure drop per unit length is proportional to the resistance per unit length of vessel. From Poiseuille's law (which will yield a crude estimate of the relations among ΔP, Q, and vessel dimensions), we would expect that a reduction in radius (r) to one-half of normal would produce a sixteenfold increase in resistance, and hence in ΔP (because R is inversely proportional to r^4). Thus the pressure drop across the narrowed arterial segment would be 16 x 0.1, or 1.6, mm Hg. Therefore, such a restriction in the arterial lumen would be expected to have only a negligible effect on blood flow to the myocardium supplied by that vessel. (See pp. 441-443 in *Physiology* 3rd ed.)

3. If the radius of the atherosclerotic segment were reduced to one-fourth, rather than to one-half, of normal, the consequence would be much more pronounced. Again, if we assume that Poiseuille's law applies, a reduction in radius to one-fourth of normal would increase the resistance by a factor of 256 (i.e., 4^4). Thus if the flow were unchanged from the preceding example, the pressure drop across the narrowed segment would now be 256 x 0.01, or 25.6, mm Hg; that is, the downstream pressure would be 25.6 mm Hg less than the upstream pressure. This diminished pressure distal to the lesion would be the pressure available for perfusing the myocardial vascular bed supplied by the left circumflex coronary artery. Hence, such a vascular lesion would be associated with a reduced blood supply to the perfused myocardium. Furthermore, slight additional narrowings of the affected vascular segment would evoke disproportionately greater curtailments of blood flow. (See pp. 441-443 in *Physiology* 3rd ed.)

4. The total peripheral resistance (TPR) of the adult was (95-5)/5 = 18 mm Hg/L/min, and that of the baby was (95-5)/1 = 90 mm Hg/L/min. (See pp. 443-446 in *Physiology* 3rd ed.)

5. The TPR of the baby is so much greater than that of the adult because the baby has a much smaller number of parallel resistance vessels (mainly arterioles) than does the adult. Therefore the same pressure gradient (90 mm Hg) from the aorta to the right atrium is able to force a blood flow of only 1 L/min through the systemic resistance vessels in the baby, whereas that same pressure gradient forces 5 L/min to flow through the much larger number of parallel resistance vessels in the adult. (See pp. 443-446 in *Physiology* 3rd ed.)

CHAPTER 27

Case 1

1. The mean arterial pressures were the same in both individuals, despite the differences in arterial compliance. Because both people had cardiac outputs (Q_h) of 4.8 L/min, the flow (peripheral runoff, Q_r) from arteries to veins through the systemic resistance vessels also had to be 4.8 L/min under steady state conditions. To force the flow of 4.8 L/min through a total peripheral resistance (R_t) of 20 mm Hg/L/min, the mean arteriovenous pressure difference ($P_a - P_v$) over the entire time of a cardiac cycle would have to be R_t x Q_r (or 20 x 4.8), which equals 96 mm Hg; this computation is based on the definition of total peripheral resistance (R_t), namely that $R_t = (P_a - P_v)/Q_r$. Because P_v is usually slightly greater than 0, P_a will be only slightly less than 96 mm Hg. This means arterial pressure will be independent of the arterial compliance. (See p. 459 in *Physiology* 3rd ed.)

2. The aorta was normally compliant in the younger man. This person's left ventricle ejected a stroke volume of 80 ml in 0.3 sec. Because his aorta was so distensible, most of the ejected blood could be stored in the aorta during the ejection period itself, and only a relatively small fraction of the stroke volume would pass from the arteries through the small resistance vessels and into the veins during systole (which usually occupies only a small fraction of the cardiac cycle). The remainder of the stored blood that had been ejected from the left ventricle traverses the resistance vessels throughout diastole. If the maximum increment in blood volume (ΔV_a) in the aorta during the ejection phase of systole was about 60 ml, and if the arterial compliance (C_a) of the grandson were 3 ml/mm Hg, then the change in arterial pressure (ΔP_a) during ejection would be $\Delta Va_a/C_a$ (or 60/3), which equals 20 mm Hg. Thus, at the very beginning of the period of ventricular ejection, P_a would be at its minimum value (defined as the *diastolic* arterial pressure), and as the blood accumulates in the arterial system during ejection, Pa rises to its maximum value (defined as the *systolic* arterial pressure) at some time during ejection. The diastolic pressure (P_d) would be below the mean arterial pressure and the systolic pressure (P_s) would be above the mean pressure. However, the difference between P_s and P_d, namely the *pulse pressure*, would be determined by the maximum increment in arterial volume (ΔV_a) during ventricular ejection and by the arterial compliance (C_a). (See pp. 408-410 in *Physiology* 3rd ed.)

    Similarly, the father's arterial pulse pressure is determined by the same factors. In this old person, however, the arterial system was not very compliant. Therefore, very little of the stroke volume, ejected during systole, could be stored in the arteries and thereby provide a relatively steady blood flow throughout diastole. Instead, almost the entire stroke volume had to be forced through the microcirculation during the brief period of ejection (about 0.3 sec in this example). To achieve a flow of almost 80 ml per 0.3 sec (or 240 ml/sec over this brief period) through a peripheral resistance of 20 mm Hg/L/min, the left ventricle would be required to develop a systolic pressure of almost 290 mm Hg. Furthermore, once ejection ceases, a very small translocation of blood from arteries to veins early in diastole results in a precipitous drop in pressure because the arteries are so rigid. Hence, the diastolic arterial pressure is very low, and the arterial pulse pressure is extremely large. Ordinarily, of course, such a high systolic arterial pressure is dangerous, and could not be sustained for very long. Various changes in hemodynamics (in heart rate, stroke volume, duration of systole, total peripheral resistance, and blood volume) and in the structural characteristics of the heart and arterial system take place during aging, and they enable the heart to adapt to the less compliant arterial system. (See p. 461 in *Physiology* 3rd ed.)

3. The amount of work done by the hearts of those two individuals to eject the same stroke volume (80 ml) differs markedly. The work done per beat can be estimated by multiplying the stroke volume by the mean pressure that exists during ejection. For the younger man, the stroke work is approximately

80 ml x 95 mm Hg or 7.6 L · mm Hg. For the father, on the other hand, the stroke work would be 80 ml x 290 mm Hg, or 23.2 L · mm Hg. Therefore this example shows that considerable more work must be done by the heart to force a given flow through the same total peripheral resistance when the systemic arteries are almost noncompliant than when they are very compliant. (See pp. 453-454 in *Physiology* 3rd ed.)

Case 2

1. The cardiac output (Q_h) and total peripheral resistance (R_t) in this example were not affected by the pacing frequency. The mean arterial pressure ($\overline{P}_a$) can be determined from the definition of total peripheral resistance (R_t); that is, $R_t = \overline{P}_a - P_v)/Q_h$. Thus, $\overline{P}_a - P_v = R_t \cdot Q_h$, which equals 20 x 4.8 = 96 mm Hg, regardless of the pacing frequency. Because P_v is usually only slightly greater than 0, $\overline{P}_a$ is essentially the product of peripheral resistance and cardiac output (in this case, about 96 mm Hg). Any change in cardiac output will evoke a proportionate change in $\overline{P}_a$, regardless of whether that change in cardiac output was achieved by a change in stroke volume, in heart rate, or in both. (See pp. 457-459 in *Physiology* 3rd ed.)

2. While the left ventricle is ejecting blood into a normally distensible aorta during systole, some blood is continually running out of the arteries, traversing the resistance vessels, and entering the veins. At any time during ventricular ejection, the increment in arterial volume equals the disparity between the volume of blood already ejected by the ventricle into the arteries and the amount of "peripheral runoff" from the arteries through the microcirculation and into the veins. During the initial phase of ejection (the rapid ejection phase), the rate of ejection exceeds the rate of runoff, and arterial volume (and hence also arterial pressure) progressively increases. During the secondary phase of ejection (the reduced ejection phase), the rate of runoff exceeds the rate of ejection, and arterial volume (and hence also arterial pressure) progressively decreases. (See pp. 408-410 in *Physiology* 3rd ed.)

    The volume of blood in the arteries just before ventricular ejection is the minimum arterial volume; it is this blood volume that determines the diastolic arterial pressure (P_d). During ventricular ejection, the maximum increase in arterial volume above this minimum volume may be called the *maximum volume increment* (ΔV_a). The maximum arterial volume, which prevails at the end of the rapid ejection phase of ventricular systole, accounts for the systolic arterial pressure (P_s), and the maximum volume increment (ΔV_a) accounts for the pulse pressure ($P_s - P_d$). For a given arterial compliance (C_a), the relation between ($P_s - P_d$) and ΔV_a is ($P_s - P_d$) = $\Delta V_a/C_a$.

    During pacing at a heart rate of 60 beats/min, the patient's stroke volume was 80 ml, whereas when the pacing rate was increased to 100 beats/min, the stroke volume decreased to 48 ml. A ventricular ejection of 80 ml would be expected to induce a substantially larger arterial volume increment than would a ventricular ejection of only 48 ml. Hence, the stroke volume of 80 ml would be expected to elicit a substantially greater pulse pressure than would a stroke volume of 48 ml. Because the mean arterial pressures were shown above to be equal at the two pacing rates, the arterial pressure characteristics during pacing at the slower rate would be characterized by a lower diastolic pressure and a higher systolic pressure than would prevail during pacing at the faster rate. (See pp. 460-461 in *Physiology* 3rd ed.)

Case 3

1. The equation that defines total peripheral resistance (R_t) is $R_t = (\overline{P}_a - P_v)/Q_r$. Under steady state conditions, the peripheral runoff (Q_r) and cardiac output (Q_h) are equal. If we substitute Q_h for Q_r in the above equation, and solve that equation for $\overline{P}_a$, we find:

$$\overline{P}_a = (Q_h \cdot R_t) + P_v$$

Thus mean arterial pressure depends on cardiac output, peripheral resistance, and central venous pressure. In this patient, however, cardiac output and central venous pressure were normal (and the latter is ordinarily very small compared to $\overline{P}_a$). Therefore by exclusion, the significant hemodynamic factor responsible for the patient's elevated mean arterial pressure is the high total peripheral resistance. Clinically most patients with essential hypertension, which is the most common variety of hypertension, do have an elevated peripheral resistance and a normal or slightly reduced cardiac output. (See pp. 459-462 in *Physiology* 3rd ed.)

2. The arterial pulse pressure reflects the relationship between the arterial distensibility and the disparity between the volume of blood ejected into the systemic arteries during the rapid ejection phase of systole and the volume that runs out of the arteries through the microcirculation during the same phase of the cardiac cycle. We can refer to this disparity between the input and output of blood during this brief time interval as the arterial "volume increment," ΔV_a. The "pressure increment" during a cardiac cycle is the arterial pulse pressure, by definition. From the definition of arterial compliance (C_a), the arterial pulse pressure (P_s - P_d) is related to the arterial compliance and the volume increment as follows:

$$P_s - P_d = \Delta V_a / C_a$$

Thus P_s - P_d is directly proportional to the volume increment and inversely proportional to the arterial compliance. In general, ΔV_a varies directly as the stroke volume. This patient had a normal stroke volume, and therefore we may presume that ΔV_a was also normal. Similarly, the distensibility of the patient's arterial system was normal for her age. Presumably, a normal ΔV_a imposed on a normal C_a would result in a normal arterial pulse pressure. The key to understanding why the patient had a pulse pressure of 80 mm Hg (twice the normal value of about 40 mm Hg) is that the arterial compliance varies as a function of the transmural pressure within the arteries. When we increase the pressure by adding fluid (gas or liquid) to a partially filled balloon, we find that the distensibility (compliance) of the balloon tends to decrease as we overdistend it. It takes a greater and greater increment of pressure to force a given additional volume into the balloon. A similar pressure-volume relationship exists for the arteries. As the arteries are progressively distended with blood, they become progressively less compliant as the pressure rises above normal. This tendency is exaggerated with advancing age.

Therefore in hypertensive patients, if the arterial compliance did not change with the arterial distending pressure and if the stroke volume (and presumably the volume increment) were normal, the pulse pressure would not be appreciably different regardless of whether the patient's arterial pressure was normal or elevated. However, if the arterial compliance diminishes substantially with distending pressure, then a given stroke volume (and volume increment) would be associated with a much greater pulse pressure when the arterial blood pressure was elevated than when the arterial blood pressure was normal. (See pp. 460-462 in *Physiology* 3rd ed.)

CHAPTER 28

1. The patient appears slightly cyanotic because blood in the microvessels of the skin is not fully oxygenated; this is caused in part by greater extraction of oxygen by the tissues secondary to a low blood flow (reduced cardiac output) and also to incomplete oxygenation of blood in the lungs because of edema and the consequent interference with oxygen diffusion from alveoli to capillaries. (See pp. 465 and 519 in *Physiology* 3rd ed.)

2. The neck veins are distended because of an elevated central venous pressure. This venous pressure increase is in part caused by the increased resistance to flow through the heart at the mitral valve but more importantly to the large blood volume in the vascular system. (See pp. 407 and 499 in *Physiology* 3rd ed.)

3. The blood volume is increased because of enhanced retention of sodium and water by the kidneys. With a reduced cardiac output and a consequent reduction in renal blood flow and glomerular filtration rate (GFR) by renal arteriolar constriction, excretion of electrolytes and water is diminished. The reduced GFR induces renin release; this leads to the formation of angiotensin, which enhances aldosterone release, and the latter increases the reabsorption of sodium. (See pp. 489 and 966-969 in *Physiology* 3rd ed.)

4. The velocity of peripheral blood flow is decreased in this patient because of the low cardiac output, the low blood pressure, and the compensatory arteriolar constriction. (See p. 465 in *Physiology* 3rd ed.)

5. Capillary blood flow is regulated primarily by the contractile state of the cognate arterioles. In this patient there is arteriolar constriction but also an increase in venous pressure, so the pressure gradient across the capillary beds is reduced. (See pp. 465-472 in *Physiology* 3rd ed.)

6. The venous pressure in the legs is greatly elevated because of the hypervolemia. Despite the large transmural pressure across the capillary walls, the capillaries do not rupture becaue their small diameter allows them to withstand the high intravascular pressure. According to the Laplace equation, T = pr, where T is wall tension, p is transmural pressure, and r is vessel radius. Because r is so small in the capillaries, the wall tension will not be excessive even when P is elevated. (See p. 466 in *Physiology* 3rd ed.)

7. The increased intravascular pressure tends to stretch the arterioles, especially in the feet when the individual is erect. The arteriolar transmural pressure is elevated, and this elicits contraction of the arteriolar vascular smooth muscle by a myogenic mechanism. (See p. 481 in *Physiology* 3rd ed.)

8. The endothelium plays a role in the regulation of peripheral resistance (in this patient and in normal individuals) by releasing nitric oxide (a vascular smooth muscle relaxant) in response to a variety of physiologic stimuli. (See p. 467 in *Physiology* 3rd ed.)

9. The rales heard at the lung bases are attributable to fluid in the small bronchi (and alveoli) and indicate some pulmonary edema. Fluid in the alveoli can interfere with gas exchange in the lung (especially with O_2) and the amount of oxygen taken up by the blood in the lungs. (See p. 474 in *Physiology* 3rd ed.)

10. The pulmonary edema is caused by the high pulmonary capillary pressure, which is attributable to the narrowed mitral valve. The left atrial pressure is high because of this valve lesion and because of the pressure generated by the hypertrophied left atrium in response to the obstruction. This high pressure is transmitted back to the pulmonary vasculature and can be assessed with a catheter threaded into a small pulmonary artery via a peripheral vein. (See p. 474 in *Physiology* 3rd ed.)

11. The patient has peripheral edema and ascites because the high hydrostatic pressure in the capillaries exceeds the oncotic pressure and results in capillary filtration into the tissues and abdominal cavity. The dependent parts of the body (ankles during standing and sacral region during bed rest) have the highest hydrostatic pressure and hence the greatest amount of edema. (See pp. 472-473 and 527 in *Physiology* 3rd ed.)

12. No. Water and sodium readily diffuse across capillary membranes in either direction, regardless of the presence of edema. (See p. 470 in *Physiology* 3rd ed.)

13. O_2 and CO_2 exchange in the peripheral tissue is normal because of the high diffusibility of these gases. However, in the lungs where the alveoli and small bronchi are filled with fluid, oxygen diffusion will be impaired. (See p. 471 in *Physiology* 3rd ed.)

14. Plasma protein levels in this patient are probably normal; hence, the oncotic pressure is also probably normal. If there is some degree of liver failure caused by liver congestion plus some dilution by excessive water retention, the plasma albumin levels could be below normal. (See p. 472 in *Physiology* 3rd ed.)

15. If all the capillaries were open, the surface area for capillary filtration would be increased, and edema would become more severe. When tissue pressure reaches levels that equal capillary hydrostatic pressure minus plasma oncotic pressure, the edema formation will cease. (See pp. 328 and 474 in *Physiology* 3rd ed.)

16. The movement of large molecules between blood and tissue would be slowed by the edema, which increases the diffusion distance between capillaries and parenchymal cells. Some large molecules are transported by pinocytosis, and this process would also be slowed by transport across edematous tissue. (See p. 475 in *Physiology* 3rd ed.)

17. The lymphatic vessels carry tissue fluid and extravascular plasma proteins back to the blood stream and hence tend to correct the edema. However, obstruction of lymphatics or (as in the case of this patient) high venous pressure increases edema formation. (See p. 475 in *Physiology* 3rd ed.)

18. The heart sounds are irregular because the patient has atrial fibrillation. In this condition (common in mitral stenosis with a hypertrophied and dilated left atrium) many of the aberrant electrical impulses arising in the atrium reach the ventricles when the ventricles are in a refractory state and hence do not elicit a ventricular contraction. Atrial impulses bombard the AV node and because of its long refractory period, the impulses get through at irregular intervals. (See pp. 393 and 412 in *Physiology* 3rd ed.)

19. Because many of the atrial impulses reach the ventricles during different times in their cycle, impulses that reach the ventricles when they are only partially filled, yet not refractory, will elicit a weak contraction. If the ventricles are only slightly filled when contraction occurs, the left ventricular contraction may not develop enough pressure to force open the aortic valve, and hence not eject any blood. When this occurs, sounds will be heard at the cardiac apex, but no pulse will be felt at the wrist. (See p. 393 in *Physiology* 3rd ed.)

CHAPTER 29

1. In the normal person, resistance to blood flow is greatest in the arterioles (resistance vessels). However, in this patient the large arteries are severely blocked by disease, whereas the arterioles are probably maximally dilated because of the release of vasodilator metabolites from the muscle as a result of inadequate blood supply. (See p. 478 in *Physiology* 3rd ed.)

2. The vascular smooth muscle of the arteries is damaged by the disease process, but the smooth muscle of the arterioles is functional but relaxed because of the presence of vasodilator metabolites. (See p. 478 in *Physiology* 3rd ed.)

3. The arterioles of this patient would constrict in response to stimulation of the sympathetic nerve fibers to the legs, and they would also constrict in response to norepinephrine, which is the neurohumor released by the sympathetic nerve endings in the blood vessels. (See p. 484 in *Physiology* 3rd ed.)

4. Calcium is the ion of greatest importance in contraction of vascular smooth muscle, just as it is for other smooth muscle and for skeletal and cardiac muscle. (See pp. 478-480 in *Physiology* 3rd ed.)

5. Autoregulation of blood flow refers to the constancy of blood flow in the face of changes in perfusion pressure. In this patient, autoregulation would not operate because the resistance vessels are maximally dilated, even when the arterial pressure is high because the blockage of the leg arteries impairs blood flow. (See p. 481 in *Physiology* 3rd ed.)

6. The myogenic mechanism is most important in the lower extremities, because the arteriolar constriction in response to the large hydrostatic (transmural) pressure (blood pressure plus effects of gravity in the standing position) prevents very high pressure in the leg capillaries and thereby prevents excessive capillary filtration (edema). In this patient, the myogenic mechanism would be overridden by the metabolic dilation. (See pp. 481-482 in *Physiology* 3rd ed.)

7. When stimulated by such agents as acetylcholine or ATP or by shear stress, the endothelium can synthesize and release nitric oxide, which is a potent vasodilator. In this patient, this could occur in the undamaged sections of the large arteries and in the arterioles and capillaries. (See pp. 467 and 480 in *Physiology* 3rd ed.)

8. With moderate walking, the leg muscles' need for oxygen is increased, but the blood supply, and hence the oxygen supply, is limited by the arterial obstruction. Thus ischemia of the muscle occurs and elicits pain. The substance responsible for the pain is not known, but some evidence suggests it is bradykinin and/or adenosine. (See p. 484 in *Physiology* 3rd ed.)

9. Metabolic regulation of blood flow is the adjustment of blood flow to the metabolic (oxygen) requirements of the tissue. Such regulation is mediated by release of endogenous vasodilator metabolites, such as adenosine. In this patient, the mechanism is operating continuously; that is, the inadequate blood flow causes vasodilator release and maximally dilated arterioles. (See p. 483 in *Physiology* 3rd ed.)

10. Basal tone in arterioles is partial contraction, independent of the nerves. Active hyperemia is vasodilation in response to increased metabolic activity, whereas reactive hyperemia is vasodilation that occurs after release of occlusion of an artery. In this patient, basal tone would be abolished by the metabolites, and because the arterioles are already maximally dilated (even at rest), increased

162

muscle activity or arterial occlusion could not dilate them further. (See pp. 483-484 in *Physiology* 3rd ed.)

11. Normally, the sympathetic nerves exert a tonic effect on the resistance vessels and can constrict these vessels when the nerves are reflexly activated. In this patient, there would be little if any tonic action and a limited reflex constriction because of the overriding metabolic effects. (See p. 484 in *Physiology* 3rd ed.)

12. Capacitance vessels are more sensitive to sympathetic nerve stimulation than are resistance vessels, but capacitance vessels do not respond well to metabolites, whereas resistance vessels do. In this patient, the resistance vessels would be even less sensitive to sympathetic nerve stimulation because of the predominance of the metabolic vasodilation. (See p. 485 in *Physiology* 3rd ed.)

13. Sympathetic denervation would not be of much help because sympathetic tone has been overridden by the action of the vasodilator metabolites. (See p. 484 in *Physiology* 3rd ed.)

14. A peripheral vasodilator would decrease arterial blood pressure and increase venous pressure (shift of blood from arterial to venous side of the circulation). Heart rate would reflexly increase via the baroreceptor reflex. The reduced blood pressure would make the leg symptoms worse by reducing an already inadequate blood flow. (See pp. 483, 486, and 516 in *Physiology* 3rd ed.)

15. A peripheral constrictor would exaggerate the symptoms by constricting the arterioles of the leg. This would in part be compensated by the elevated arterial blood pressure caused by constriction of resistance vessels in other parts of the body. Heart rate would decrease reflexly in response to the increased blood pressure. (See pp. 484 and 486 in *Physiology* 3rd ed.)

16. In the short term, the baroreceptor reflex keeps the blood pressure fairly constant, whereas in the long term, the adjustments in salt and water excretion (and hence blood volume) by the kidneys are of paramount importance in the regulation of blood pressure. These mechanisms also operate in this patient. (See p. 489 in *Physiology* 3rd ed.)

17. Inhalation of CO_2 would (1) increase the rate and depth of respiration by stimulation of the chemoreceptors, (2) increase blood pressure by stimulation of the vasoconstrictor center in the medulla, and (3) have little reflex effect on the leg blood flow because of the local metabolites. (See p. 490 in *Physiology* 3rd ed.)

18. In response to hypoxia, (1) respiration would increase by stimulation of the peripheral chemoreceptors (carotid and aortic bodies), (2) blood pressure would probably not change or would increase slightly, and (3) leg blood flow would be unchanged. (See p. 490 in *Physiology* 3rd ed.)

19. In the normal person at rest, neural regulation of muscle blood flow predominates, but with exercise, the local factors supervene. In this patient the local factors predominate at rest and during exercise. (See p. 491 in *Physiology* 3rd ed.)

CHAPTER 30

1. Ventricular fibrillation is a grave rhythm disturbance in which many reentry circuits proceed haphazardly throughout the ventricles. Because the myriad myocardial cells that comprise the ventricles are contracting and relaxing so asynchronously, the heart pumps no blood. In this patient, the arterial and central venous pressures were normal just before the onset of fibrillation. Therefore at the very beginning of the arrhythmia, the flow from the systemic arteries to the systemic veins through the capillaries was normal initially, even though cardiac output suddenly became zero. However, the flow through the capillaries from arteries to veins caused the arterial pressure to fall rapidly and the venous pressure to rise. This process continued until pressures equilibrated throughout the systemic vascular bed. (See pp. 494-498 in *Physiology* 3rd ed.)

2. When cardiac output suddenly became zero, blood continued to flow from arteries to veins until the pressures equilibrated. The volume of blood lost from the arteries was virtually equal to the volume of blood gained by the veins (i.e., $\Delta V_a \cong \Delta V_v$). If the arterial and venous compliances were equal, then the decline in arterial pressure would have been equal to the rise in venous pressure.

    From the definition of compliance, we can predict the changes in arterial and venous pressure that take place when a given volume of blood is translocated from the arteries to the veins. By rearranging the definitions of C_a and C_v:

    $$\Delta P_a = \Delta V_a / C_a$$

    $$\Delta P_v = \Delta V_v / C_v$$

    However, because $\Delta V_a = - \Delta V_v$, it follows that:

    $$C_a \cdot \Delta P_a = - C_v \cdot \Delta P_v$$

    Therefore

    $$\Delta P_v / \Delta P_a = - C_a / C_v$$

    That is, the ratio of the increment in P_v to the decrement in P_a is inversely proportional to their respective compliances. Thus if their compliances were equal, then the fall in P_a would equal the rise in P_v. However, the veins are much more compliant than the arteries, and the compliance ratio is about 20 to 1. Therefore the decline in systemic arterial pressure is about 20 times greater than the rise in systemic venous pressure when the heart stops beating. (See pp. 494-498 in *Physiology* 3rd ed.)

3. One manifestation of an enhancement of myocardial contractility is that for a given ventricular filling pressure (which, for the right ventricle, is equivalent to the central venous pressure), the heart will pump a greater cardiac output. If this new drug has no direct effect on the resistance blood vessels, an increase in cardiac output will tend to redistribute the blood volume such that a greater fraction will reside in the arteries and a smaller fraction will reside in the veins. This will be reflected by a rise in arterial blood pressure and a fall in central venous pressure. (See pp. 494-499 in *Physiology* 3rd ed.)

4. According to the Frank-Starling mechanism, cardiac performance (including cardiac output) varies as a function of the initial length of the myocardial fibers (as determined by the filling pressure). For a given level of contractility, the Frank-Starling mechanism can be represented by a curve of cardiac

output (Y axis) as a function of the ventricular filling pressure (X axis). When contractility is enhanced, however, the characteristic curve is shifted to the left; thus the Frank-Starling mechanism is actually represented by a family of curves, rather than by a single curve. A pure increase in myocardial contractility will cause the coordinates of the operating point to shift upward and to the left from the control contractility curve to the enhanced contractility curve. This diagonal shift will reflect the *increase* in cardiac output and the *decrease* in central venous pressure. The precise diagonal path from one curve to the other is dictated by the specific "vascular function curve" that defines the state of the vascular system—that is, the curve depends on the total blood volume, the total peripheral resistance, and the arterial and venous compliances. (See pp. 502-503 in *Physiology* 3rd ed.)

5. When a recumbent person assumes the upright posture, gravity tends to redistribute the blood volume toward those vessels that lie below the heart. The pressure in the blood vessels below the heart (the "dependent" vessels) tends to rise as a function of the distance (h) below the heart; the increase in pressure (ΔP) equals $h\rho g$, where ρ is the density of blood, and g is the acceleration of gravity. Because the veins are more compliant than the arteries, most of the increased blood volume resides in the dependent veins. With respect to the magnitude of the cardiac filling pressure, this sequestration of blood volume in the dependent veins has an influence on cardiac output and mean arterial pressure similar to that exerted by blood loss from the body. (See pp. 505-507 in *Physiology* 3rd ed.)

6. The tendency for gravity to reduce cardiac output and arterial blood pressure when an individual shifts from the recumbent to the upright position quickly invokes the baroreceptor reflexes. As the pressure decreases in the carotid sinuses and aortic arch, the changes in baroreceptor activity in these regions bring about increases in total peripheral resistance, in heart rate, and in myocardial contractility. These responses tend to minimize the reductions in arterial blood pressure and in cerebral blood flow (which accounts for the light-headedness). Another compensatory reaction involves an increase in skeletal muscle activity; as a person becomes light-headed, he or she tends to move more. Contraction of the muscles in the legs (acting in conjunction with the valves in the leg veins) tends to massage blood (an auxiliary pump) in the leg veins back toward the heart. (See pp. 506-507 and 520 in *Physiology* 3rd ed.)

7. The major component of the baroreceptor reflexes in buffering the tendency for the arterial blood pressure to fall when an individual assumes the upright posture is the increase in total peripheral resistance, which is achieved by a contraction of the smooth muscle in arterioles throughout the body. The use of a vascular smooth muscle relaxant, for example, in the treatment of hypertension, would tend to prevent an effective increase in total peripheral resistance and would thereby attenuate substantially the efficacy of the baroreceptor reflexes to buffer a reduction in arterial blood pressure. (See p. 506 in *Physiology* 3rd ed.)

8. Cardiac output (Q_h) equals stroke volume (SV) times heart rate (HR). When the pacing rate was 60 beats/min, Q_h was 80 x 60, or 4800 ml/min. When the pacing rate was 100 beats/min, Q_h was 48 x 100, or 4800 ml/min. Hence Q_h was equal at these two pacing rates. (See pp. 475 and 495 in *Physiology* 3rd ed.)

9. An increase in HR tends to increase Q_h, but it also abridges the time available for ventricular filling. Thus over a substantial range of heart rates, SV tends to be inversely proportional to HR. Therefore over that range of heart rates, Q_h is not appreciably affected by changes in HR. At heart rates below this plateau range, further reductions in HR are not attended by proportionate increases in diastolic filling volumes, because the ventricles are approaching their maximal volumes (partly imposed by the pericardium). Hence, Q_h decreases sharply with further reductions in HR. At the other end of the frequency range, additional increases in HR do not allow sufficient time for adequate ventricular

filling. Hence, the curtailed filling volumes are not compensated for by the increased number of cardiac contractions per minute. Therefore, Q_h decreases sharply with further increases in HR. (See pp. 504-505 in *Physiology* 3rd ed.)

CHAPTER 31

1. An intravenous infusion of adenosine dilates arterioles, particularly in the heart. In cases where coronary artery obstruction exists and hence blood flow is limited, the arterioles distal to the obstructed vessels become maximally dilated by the release of local metabolites (e.g., adenosine) and cannot be dilated further by the administered adenosine. However, the cognate arterioles of the patent arteries dilate. As a result, the pressure in these patent arteries decreases, and flow from these arteries via collateral vessels to the ischemic myocardium is reduced. This produces greater myocardial ischemia with precordial pain and/or electrocardiographic evidence of ischemia. With this type of stress test, the heart is stressed by reducing its oxygen supply rather than by increasing the cardiac workload with exercise. (See p. 516 in *Physiology* 3rd ed.)

2. Potassium chloride was given to arrest the heart in diastole in order to make the operation technically easier and to reduce the oxygen need of the myocardium during the time when blood flow to the heart muscle and lungs is stopped. The cold saline also reduces the cardiac oxygen needs by lowering cardiac metabolic activity and thereby prevents ischemic damage to the myocardium. (See pp. 399 and 516 in *Physiology* 3rd ed.)

3. The increased aortic resistance during diastole raises blood pressure proximal to the balloon and thereby improves coronary perfusion at a time when extravascular compression by the myocardium is absent. During systole the deflation of the balloon reduces resistance to ejection by the left ventricle and thereby decreases cardiac work and the oxygen needs of the myocardium. (See p. 512 in *Physiology* 3rd ed.)

4. For measurement of coronary blood flow by thermodilution, a double lumen catheter is inserted into the coronary sinus via a peripheral vein. Ice-cold saline is injected from the catheter tip, and a temperature probe a few centimeters proximal (downstream) to the catheter tip senses the blood temperature. The smaller the temperature change after the cold saline injection, the greater the coronary sinus blood flow. (See p. 510 in *Physiology* 3rd ed.)

5. The physical factors that affect coronary blood flow in this patient are the systolic, and especially the diastolic, aortic pressure, the extravascular compression exerted by the heart muscle on the coronary vessels, blood viscosity, and of greatest importance, arterial and arteriolar resistances. (See p. 511 in *Physiology* 3rd ed.)

6. The sympathetic nerves do not play a significant role in the regulation of coronary blood flow in this patient, particularly because the arterioles are dilated by local metabolites. Even in normal individuals the local metabolic factors predominate over neural factors in the regulation of coronary blood flow. (See p. 513 in *Physiology* 3rd ed.)

7. Several agents have been proposed as mediators of the vasodilation that occurs in the coronary circulation when blood flow to the myocardium is inadequate. Adenosine is involved, and as yet unidentified substances may also contribute to vasodilation secondary to ischemia. (See p. 514 in *Physiology* 3rd ed.)

8. No. Endocardial blood flow would be more compromised than epicardial blood flow because of the greater vascular compression by the endocardial myocardium. (See p. 512 in *Physiology* 3rd ed.)

9. It is not firmly established how nitroglycerin relieves angina pectoris, but evidence suggests that (1) it dilates coronary collateral vessels and (2) it decreases preload by relaxing the large veins such as the vena cava. The drug dilates resistance vessels throughout the body and thereby produces a transient reduction in arterial blood pressure. (See p. 516 in *Physiology* 3rd ed.)

10. The progressive narrowing of a coronary artery results in the development of collateral vessels from patent coronary artery, which supplies some blood to the muscle served by the obstructed artery. The collaterals develop from preexisting capillaries, and the combination of ischemia and the high pressure gradient leads to collateral vessel formation. (See p. 515 in *Physiology* 3rd ed.)

11. Relative to other tissues, the vascular beds of the heart and especially the brain are not very responsive to general sympathetic activation. These two vascular beds are primarily under the control of local metabolic factors. Skin, gastrointestinal tract, kidney, and resting skeletal muscle show a high degree of vasoconstriction in response to sympathetic activity. However, in contracting skeletal muscle sympathetic neural regulation yields to local metabolic factors. (See pp. 513, 518, 520, 523, 525, and 527 in *Physiology* 3rd ed.)

12. An increase in environmental temperature would dilate skin blood vessels, which facilitates heat loss and tends to maintain a constant core temperature. This dilation would decrease vascular resistance and could decrease arterial blood pressure, especially if body temperature rises and other vascular beds also dilate. If body temperature is increased, an added burden is placed on the heart and circulation by increasing the oxygen demands of the myocardium and other body tissues. (See p. 518 in *Physiology* 3rd ed.)

13. Cold exposure would constrict the skin arterioles, thereby preventing heat loss and maintaining body temperature constant. This vasoconstriction is accomplished via a skin reflex and via cooled blood reaching the temperature-regulating center in the hypothalamus. Blood pressure could be reflexly increased by cold exposure. Any reduction in body temperature would reduce the metabolic needs of the body an thereby reduce the heart and body oxygen requirements. (See p. 518 in *Physiology* 3rd ed.)

14. The venous valves in this patient (and in all subjects) serve to aid in the return of blood to the heart. With the patient in the upright position, muscle contraction in the leg squeezes the veins and forces blood out of them in the direction of the heart, because the venous valves prevent flow in the opposite direction. (See p. 520 in *Physiology* 3rd ed.)

15. The pain in the right leg (caused by ischemia) produces vasodilation in the contralateral sensory-motor cortex in the region that serves the leg. This response is probably mediated by the release of nitric oxide from the endothelium of the vessels in this cortical region and is not associated with adenosine release in the cortex. Adenosine release is associated with either increased metabolic activity or a reduced oxygen supply. (See p. 523 in *Physiology* 3rd ed.)

16. With physical exercise, blood flow is increased to the active muscles by the action of local metabolites, and it is decreased to the gastrointestinal tract and liver by arteriolar constriction mediated by the sympathetic nerves. (See pp. 515, 527, and 533 in *Physiology* 3rd ed.)

17. Cerebral blood flow in this patient and in normal individuals is increased by CO_2 inhalation. Because the cerebral arterioles are probably somewhat dilated as a result of the carotid artery atherosclerosis and the consequent increase in resistance to blood flow, CO_2 would have less effect in this patient than in a normal person. (See p. 523 in *Physiology* 3rd ed.)

18. Hypoxia would increase cerebral blood flow by enhancing the formation and release of adenosine and other vasodilator metabolites in the brain tissue. (See p. 524 in *Physiology* 3rd ed.)

19. The atherosclerosis reduces blood flow to the brain and can cause brief reversible "strokes" called transient ischemic attacks (TIAs). Arteriolar resistance would be reduced because of the release of vasodilator metabolites from the inadequately perfused brain tissue. (See p. 523 in *Physiology* 3rd ed.)

20. A patent ductus arteriosus causes a continuous murmur over the precordium because of blood flow from the aorta (higher pressure) to the pulmonary artery (lower pressure). The murmur is loudest during systole, when the pressure gradient between the aorta and pulmonary artery is greatest. (See p. 527 in *Physiology* 3rd ed.)

CHAPTER 32

Case 1

1. In anticipation of a race, the runner's sympathetic nervous system is activated (central command), and catecholamines are released from the adrenal medulla. This results in cardiac acceleration, increased myocardial contractility, increased cardiac output, peripheral vasoconstriction, and an increase in blood pressure. (See p. 532 in *Physiology* 3rd ed.)

2. Heart rate continues to increase during the exercise, until the rate reaches a plateau of about 180 beats/min at maximum effort. Peripheral resistance decreases because of relaxation of arterioles in active muscle and skin (as body temperature rises). Skin blood flow increases, which aids in heat loss. Blood flow to inactive muscle, kidney, and gastrointestinal tract is reduced. (See p. 534 in *Physiology* 3rd ed.)

3. The increased production of CO_2 by the active muscles is removed in the lungs by the greater depth and rate of respiration, and therefore arterial PCO_2 ($PaCO_2$) remains normal. (See p. 492 in *Physiology* 3rd ed.)

4. Blood flow to the leg muscles increases because of local factors, which include the release of vasodilator metabolites (e.g., adenosine), the increase in muscle temperature, and the local decrease in pH (increased CO_2 and lactic acid). The arterioles dilate and more capillaries open (capillary recruitment). (See pp. 521 and 535 in *Physiology* 3rd ed.)

5. Interstitial pressure in the active muscles increases because of movement of fluid from the vascular compartment to the interstitial space. The greater hydrostatic pressure (increase in blood pressure plus arteriolar dilation) enhances capillary filtration, until the increase in tissue pressure counterbalances the elevated intracapillary pressure. (See p. 534 in *Physiology* 3rd ed.)

6. Oxygen extraction from the blood perfusing the active muscles is increased, and therefore venous blood oxygen content is reduced. However, the enhanced respiratory activity results in normal oxygenation of the blood in the lungs and hence a normal arterial oxygen content. (See p. 535 in *Physiology* 3rd ed.)

7. Venous return is facilitated in running by the following: (1) sympathetic-mediated contraction of capacitance vessels, (2) muscle compression of the leg veins with one-way valves, and (3) the greater negative pressure in the thorax caused by deeper and more rapid respiration. (See pp. 520 and 534 in *Physiology* 3rd ed.)

8. In the trained athlete, stroke volume is large at rest and increases further with exercise, whereas in the untrained individual, stroke volume shows little change and heart rate increases greatly. The actual *cause* of the increase in cardiac output is the decrease in peripheral resistance. Mean arterial blood pressure increases slightly, as does pulse pressure (i.e., systolic pressure increases a little more than does diastolic pressure). (See pp. 505 and 536 in *Physiology* 3rd ed.)

9. At the start of the exercise, activation of the sympathetic nervous system causes constriction of the skin resistance vessels. As body temperature rises during the exercise, the skin vessels dilate, and therefore heat loss is facilitated. If the exercise is very severe and exhaustion occurs, the skin vessels constrict and permit more of the circulating blood to perfuse the active muscles. This skin vasoconstriction can lead to serious hyperthermia. (See p. 535 in *Physiology* 3rd ed.)

10. The limitation of performance in this runner is oxygen delivery to the active muscles. Hence, the pumping capacity of the heart is the main limiting factor. (See p. 535 in *Physiology* 3rd ed.)

Case 2

1. The body is able to mobilize a number of mechanisms to compensate for the loss of blood. The baroreceptor reflexes are probably the most important of these mechanisms. In response to blood loss, the carotid sinus and aortic arch baroreceptors signal any reduction in arterial pressure to the nucleus tractus solitarius in the medulla oblongata. This nucleus, in turn, initiates an increase in sympathetic activity to the heart and vasculature and a decrease in parasympathetic activity to the heart. These actions tend to increase cardiac output and mean arterial blood pressure. The arterial chemoreceptor and cerebral ischemia reflexes also serve to increase sympathetic neural activity to the cardiovascular system. The release of endogenous vasoconstrictor substances, notably epinephrine, vasopressin, and angiotensin, also tends to restore arterial blood pressure toward normal levels. The reduction in peripheral capillary pressure leads to a reabsorption of interstitial fluid into the vascular compartment, thereby tending to augment the total blood volume. Finally, the kidneys act to conserve fluid in response to renal vasoconstriction and to increased blood levels of vasopressin and aldosterone. (See pp. 537-540 in *Physiology* 3rd ed.)

2. Hemorrhage also sets into motion various decompensatory mechanisms that tend to aggravate the tenuous state of the cardiovascular system. The low arterial pressure induced by the blood loss serves to diminish the coronary blood flow. This curtailment of myocardial perfusion in turn may diminish cardiac output and thereby further reduce the arterial blood pressure. Other vicious cycles that may be invoked are severe depression of the central nervous system, generalized acidosis, blood-clotting aberrations, and depression of the reticuloendothelial system. All of these reactions tend to diminish the efficacy of the various compensatory mechanisms. If the decompenstory mechanisms predominate over the compensatory mechanisms, cardiovascular function will deteriorate and death will ensue. (See pp. 540-542 in *Physiology* 3rd ed.)

3. Fig. 32-1 shows hypothetical cardiac and vascular function curves for the effects of a specific, positive inotropic drug on cardiac output and central venous pressure during normovolemia, hypovolemia, and generalized vasoconstriction. Point A represents the intersection between the cardiac and vascular function curves of either soldier under normal conditions (before the injury). In such a normal individual, administration of the positive inotropic drug would increase the cardiac output and decrease the central venous pressure substantially, as reflected by the shift in intersecting points from A to B in the figure. Pure hypovolemia (in the absence of compensatory vascular reactions) would cause a parallel downward shift of the vascular function curve, as shown in the figure. The same positive inotropic drug would be expected to evoke increases in cardiac output and decreases in central P_v similar to those elicited under normovolemic conditions. Hypovolemia rapidly induces reflex vasoconstriction, however, and such vasoconstriction is reflected by a counterclockwise rotation of the vascular function curve. Under such conditions, even a substantial enhancement of myocardial contractility does not elicit a very great increase in cardiac output (as denoted by the small differences in the Y-coordinates of points *E* and *F*). The reason for the counterclockwise rotation of this curve is that when peripheral resistance is increased, a given change in cardiac output produces a greater

reduction in central P_v than it does when resistance is normal. Thus when peripheral resistance is elevated, any agent that tends to increase cardiac output would also tend to lower central P_v substantially, and this in turn would minimize the augmentation of cardiac output. (See pp. 494-505 in *Physiology* 3rd ed.)

CHAPTER 33

1. PaO$_2$ is the partial pressure of oxygen in arterial blood and is expressed in mm Hg. This pressure is exerted by oxygen molecules in their gas phase (dissolved in the plasma component of blood, as opposed to chemically combined with hemoglobin). Note that once oxygen is chemically bound with hemoglobin, it no longer exerts a pressure. Note also that PO$_2$ (without the *a*) is the generic term for partial pressure of oxygen in any gas or liquid, and it should not be used without reference to the site (e.g., inspired air, alveolar air, pulmonary veins, etc.).

    SaO$_2$ is the saturation of hemoglobin with oxygen in arterial blood, and it is expressed as a percentage of total binding sites that are combined with oxygen. Thus if 95 of every 100 hemoglobin binding sites are combined with oxygen, the blood has an SaO$_2$ of 95%. A major, but not the only, determinant of SaO$_2$ is the PaO$_2$.

    The relation between PaO$_2$ and SaO$_2$ is illustrated by the oxygen-hemoglobin equilibrium (dissociation) curve, the exact shape and position of which depend on several factors (pH; 2,3-diphosphoglycerate; PaCO$_2$; and body temperature). (See pp. 548 and 555 in *Physiology* 3rd ed.)

2. Oxygen content is a measurement of quantity. Unlike PAO$_2$ and SaO$_2$, oxygen content directly reflects the number of oxygen molecules in the blood; the units are ml O$_2$ per 100 ml, or per liter, of blood (both *per dl* and *per L* will be found in various texts and also in hospital laboratories). Neither PAO$_2$ nor SaO$_2$ gives information on the content of oxygen in the blood; they only provide a pressure and percentage of saturation, respectively. PAO$_2$ and the shape and position of the oxygen equilibrium curve determine the SaO$_2$. The SaO$_2$ and the hemoglobin (Hb) content determine the oxygen content (along with a small contribution from dissolved PaO$_2$). Clearly, without knowledge of the hemoglobin content there is no way to know *how much* oxygen is in the blood. Anemia does not affect PaO$_2$ or SaO$_2$. Hence a severely anemic patient could have a low oxygen content and a normal PaO$_2$ and SaO$_2$. Arterial oxygen content is provided by the following formula:

    (Amount O$_2$ bound to hemoglobin)   (Amount O$_2$ dissolved in blood)
    SaO$_2$ x Hb (g/dl) x 1.34 ml O$_2$/g Hb + 0.003 ml O$_2$/mm Hg PaO$_2$/dl

    Because SaO$_2$ is provided in the data given, there is no need to use the hemoglobin-oxygen equilibrium curve to answer this question. Based on these data, the patient's arterial O$_2$ content is

    0.90 x 14 g Hb/dl x 1.34 ml O$_2$/g Hb + 0.003 ml O$_2$ (60 mm Hg)/dl
    = 16.9 ml O$_2$/dl + 0.18 ml O$_2$ = 17.1 ml O$_2$/dl blood*

    *Or 171 ml O$_2$/L blood

    (See p. 556 in *Physiology* 3rd ed.)

3. Minute ventilation = respiratory rate x tidal volume = 25 breaths/min x 400 ml = 10 L/min; this value is higher than the typical resting minute ventilation of 6 L/min. Because neither dead space volume nor alveolar volume is given, we cannot calculate dead space ventilation or alveolar ventilation. Even though his respiratory rate and minute ventilation are increased, we should not state that he is hyperventilating (for the reasons explained in the next question). However, we can answer this question and assess overall adequacy of alveolar ventilation from the measured PaO$_2$ (see the next two questions). (See p. 559 in *Physiology* 3rd ed.)

4. The alveolar ventilation equation is called "the central equation of pulmonary physiology." In fact, this equation is crucial to understanding many physiologic derangements in patients with respiratory tract problems. Rearranging the equation we obtain

$$P_{ACO_2} \quad \frac{V_{CO_2} \times 0.863}{V_A}$$

Thus alveolar P_{CO_2} is directly proportional to the CO_2 production (V_{CO_2}) and inversely proportional to alveolar ventilation (V_A). Any *proportionate* changes in the V_{CO_2} and V_A will not change P_{ACO_2}; any *disproportionate* changes will affect P_{ACO_2} predictably, depending on whether the greater change is in the numerator or denominator. For example, a 40% rise in V_A and a 10% rise in V_{CO_2} will lower P_{ACO_2}. (See p. 560 in *Physiology* 3rd ed.)

5. Alveolar P_{CO_2} in the alveolar ventilation and alveolar gas equations can be replaced by the measured arterial P_{CO_2}; this is true because there is no "gradient" between the two values, as there is between alveolar and arterial P_{O_2}. Substituting P_{aCO_2} in the alveolar ventilation equation, we see that P_{aCO_2} is determined by the *ratio* of CO_2 production to alveolar ventilation:

$$P_{ACO_2} \quad \frac{V_{CO_2} \times 0.863}{V_A}$$

Normally, the amount of V_A is sufficient to excrete the produced CO_2 and thereby keep P_{aCO_2} in the normal range (36 to 44 mm Hg). With increases in CO_2 production (as during modest exercise), V_A will normally rise a proportionate amount and thereby maintain a normal P_{aCO_2}. If V_A does not rise along with V_{CO_2}, or if V_A falls while V_{CO_2} does not or if V_A falls more than V_{CO_2}, V_A will be reduced out of proportion for the V_{CO_2}; this situation represents *hypoventilation*, which raises P_{aCO_2}. Conversely, when V_A is elevated out of proportion to the V_{CO_2} there is *hyperventilation*, which reduces P_{aCO_2}. By definition, then, hyperventilation and hypoventilation refer only to a specific P_{aCO_2} value, which in turn reflects the *state of alveolar ventilation relative to CO_2 production*. Note that hyperventilation and hypoventilation do not refer to rate or depth of breathing, or a patient's respiratory effort. This is why you cannot say, from observation alone, that a patient is "hyperventilating." Irrespective of rate or depth of breathing, a patient with lung disease may in fact be hyper-, hypo-, or normally ventilating relative to CO_2 production. (See p. 559 in *Physiology* 3rd ed.)

6. From the alveolar gas equation, $P_{AO_2} = 114$ mm Hg. This patient is hyperventilating. Hence alveolar P_{O_2} is increased. (The alveolar gas equation shows that P_{AO_2} always increases if P_{aCO_2} decreases, other factors remaining unchanged.) (See p. 560 in *Physiology* 3rd ed.)

7. $P_{AO_2} - P_{aO_2} = 114 - 60 = 54$ mm Hg and is definitely abnormal; normal ($P_{AO_2} - P_{aO_2}$) for a man this age, breathing ambient air, is about 10 to 15 mm Hg. For someone who is breathing room air at sea level and who has a P_{aCO_2} of 40 mm Hg, $P_{AO_2} = 102$ mm Hg. Under the same conditions, the normal P_{aO_2} for a man this age should be about 90 mm Hg; ($P_{AO_2} - P_{aO_2}$) would then be $102 - 90 = 12$ mm Hg. Although this patient's P_{aO_2} is slightly elevated because of hyperventilation, his P_{aO_2} is reduced (their difference is 54 mm Hg). This large difference between P_{AO_2} and P_{aO_2} indicates a significant defect in getting oxygen from the alveoli into the pulmonary circulation. (See pp. 559 and 588 in *Physiology* 3rd ed.)

8. *Ventilation*: The patient is hyperventilating; in other words, his level of alveolar ventilation is more than needed to excrete his metabolic production CO_2 and to keep Pa_{CO_2} in the normal range. *Oxygenation*: First, the transfer of oxygen from alveoli into the pulmonary capillaries is impaired; this is evident because (P_{AO_2} - Pa_{O_2}) is greater than normal. Second, hemoglobin content is normal, but oxygen saturation is reduced slightly at 90%; therefore his oxygen content is also reduced. (See pp. 555-556 and 558 in *Physiology* 3rd ed.)

9. A *lung volume* is a quantity of air not subdivided further (e.g., tidal volume, residual volume). A *lung capacity* is a quantity that includes two or more lung volumes (e.g., total lung capacity, functional residual capacity). (See p. 558 in *Physiology* 3rd ed.)

10. The forced vital capacity (FVC) is slightly reduced below the lower normal limit of 80%, and the FEV-1 is reduced even more. When the FEV-1 is reduced more than FVC, there is some air flow obstruction (the patient cannot exhale forcefully at a normal rate). At the same time, the total lung capacity and residual volume are above normal; this finding suggests some air trapping. Overall, these changes are typical of obstructive airway disease commonly seen in long-term smokers. If air flow remains obstructed despite treatment, the patient is said to have chronic obstructive pulmonary disease (COPD). (See pp. 572-573 in *Physiology* 3rd ed.)

11. Total lung capacity and residual volume cannot be determined by spirometry alone. (See p. 558 in *Physiology* 3rd ed.)

CHAPTER 34

1. *Total lung capacity* (TLC) would probably be reduced. TLC is the amount of air contained within the lungs at the point of maximal inhalation. If there is something, such as edema fluid, occupying or obliterating the alveolar spaces, the volume of air at TLC probably will be lower than normal. Thus in pulmonary edema and all other space-occupying disturbances of the lungs, the TLC will be reduced.

   Surface tension would be increased. The edema fluid in the alveolar spaces washes away surfactant, the complex phospholipid that reduces surface tension at the air–alveolar wall interface. As a result, the patient's alveoli tend to collapse as she exhales, further worsening her lung compliance and overall clinical condition. (The infant respiratory distress syndrome is characterized by pulmonary edema, which is caused by lack of surfactant at birth.)

   Lung compliance would be reduced. The edema fluid not only washes away surfactant, but it also infiltrates the interstitium and makes the lungs stiffer than normal. Hence, a greater translung pressure is required to inflate them, and the patient must work harder than normal to breathe. At some point, if the pulmonary edema does not respond to treatment, the patient will tire and require mechanical ventilation (as happened to this patient).

   Her *work of breathing*, for the reasons just described, is increased.

   Airway resistance would be reduced, although less than the fall in compliance and TLC. Most of the airway resistance arises from the larger airways (i.e., those with a cross-sectional diameter greater than 2 mm). Airways less than 2 mm diameter, while more numerous than larger airways, provide only about 20% of the respiratory tract's total airway resistance. Even if these "small airways" are narrowed 50% by edema fluid, the impact on the total measured airway resistance may not be easily discernible.

   On the other hand, if edema fluid enters the interstitium surrounding the larger airways and causes them to constrict (as sometimes happens), their narrowing should cause a more obvious increase in airway resistance. Some patients with pulmonary edema actually wheeze and sound "asthmatic"; they definitely have increased airway resistance. (See pp. 563-575 in *Physiology* 3rd ed.)

2. The machine has taken over her breathing. She has a measured tidal volume of 500 ml and a translung pressure difference of 30 - 0 cm H_2O. Thoracic compliance, the change in thoracic volume over change in pressure, is 600 ml/30 cm H_2O, or 20 ml/cm H_2O. This is the compliance of her lungs and chest wall together, because the ventilator must expand both in delivering this tidal volume.

   Compliance is a measurement of how much pressure is required to overcome the elastic forces of a structure (lungs, chest wall, lungs and chest wall, etc.). If pressure is being exerted to overcome airway resistance as well, you will not obtain a true compliance measurement. For this reason, lung compliance measurements must always be made at a point of no air flow, so that airway resistance does not affect the pressure being measured. Asthma exemplifies this point. The pressure volume curve in asthma is close to normal or is shifted slightly to the left (i.e., the lungs have normal or slightly elevated compliance). If pressure to distend the lungs is measured *during* breathing (i.e., during air flow), the increased resistance of asthmatic airways will give a higher pressure than at a point of no air flow; the resulting "compliance" measurement will be artificially low, and the asthmatic patient's lungs will appear stiffer than they really are. (See pp. 564-565 in *Physiology* 3rd ed.)

176

3. Airway resistance = change in pressure over air flow. Pressure change is the difference between Pao, the airway pressure at the mouth, and PA, the alveolar pressure. Airway resistance is not easy to measure in a nonintubated patient because there is no simple way to obtain both pressures. (Airway resistance can be measured with body plethysmography.) In an intubated patient the measurement is easy to accomplish, but it will include the increased resistance of the endotracheal tube and will thereby confound the patient's true airway resistance.

    For a patient who is connected to a mechanical ventilator, Pao is the peak airway pressure measured *during* air flow. PA is obtained by briefly occluding the airway at the point of peak airway pressure (e.g., 0.5 second); during occlusion, air does not flow, and the pressure will equal PA. From the data provided,

$$\text{Raw} = \frac{\text{Pao - PA}}{\text{flow}} = \frac{35 - 25 \text{ cm H}_2\text{O}}{1 \text{ L/sec}} = \frac{10}{1} = 10 \text{ cm H}_2\text{O/L/sec}$$

    Her resistance in the airway (Raw) is elevated, but most of this elevation can be attributed to her endotracheal tube. Her true pulmonary resistance cannot be determined. (See pp. 571-572 in *Physiology* 3rd ed.)

4. a. Total lung capacity (TLC)
    b. Forced vital capacity (FVC)
    c. Residual volume (RV)
    (See p. 558 in *Physiology* 3rd ed.)

5. In the FVC maneuver, maximal air flow occurs shortly after exhalation begins, well within the first second; this fastest rate of flow is called the peak expiratory flow rate, or "peak flow." Peak flow (see Fig. 34-14 in *Physiology* 3rd ed.) is the highest point on the expiratory flow volume curve. Peak flow is dependent on the lung capacity at which the exhalation effort begins; the higher the initial lung capacity, the higher the potential peak flow. Expanding the lungs fully maximizes the cross-sectional diameter of the large airways and reduces their air flow resistance; thus peak flow exceeds that achievable at lower lung volumes. If she did not inhale maximally before commencing this maneuver, her peak flow would be less than the flow she could achieve starting from TLC. (See pp. 573-574 in *Physiology* 3rd ed.)

6. Functional residual capacity (FRC). A typical normal value for FRC is about 3.5 L.

    Intrapleural pressure at FRC is negative because, at FRC, the elastic recoil of the chest wall, which tends to expand that structure outward, is balanced by the elastic recoil of the lungs, which tends to contract them.

    If the chest wall is punctured, as long as there is a communication between the atmosphere and intrapleural space, air will rush in until the intrapleural pressure equals the atmospheric pressure. As a result, the elastic recoil of the lung on that side will no longer be opposed by the chest wall elastic recoil, and the lung will collapse. This condition is called a pneumothorax. (See pp. 558 and 567 in *Physiology* 3rd ed.)

7.

	Emphysema	Pulmonary fibrosis
Elastic recoil	D	I
Compliance	I	D
TLC	I	D
FRC	I	D
FVC	D	D
RV	I	I
$\dot{V}E$	V	V
Pa_{O_2} (rest)	V	V
Pa_{CO_2} (rest)	V	V

D = decreased, I = increased, V = variable

Emphysema is a chronic lung condition characterized by loss of alveolar-capillary membranes and supporting elastic tissue; it usually occurs from long-term cigarette smoking. The loss of elastic tissue makes the lungs more easily distensible than normal (increased compliance), and allows them to expand outward against the chest wall (increased TLC). At the same time, airways close earlier than normal during expiration and thus the FRC and RV are increased. For the same reason, FVC tends to be decreased. Minute ventilation increases as a consequence of the increase in dead space. Arterial blood gases can be normal or abnormal in emphysema. If the increased minute ventilation goes to the increased dead space *and* provides enough alveolar ventilation to wash out the patient's CO_2, Pa_{CO_2} will stay in the normal range. In advanced emphysema, however, the respiratory muscles may be too weak to perform the increased work of breathing, and Pa_{CO_2} may rise. As for Pa_{O_2}, there may be enough alveolar units with normal or near normal V/Q ratios to keep Pa_{O_2} in the normal range, at least at rest. However, in advanced stages of emphysema, V/Q imbalance may be so severe that Pa_{O_2} is reduced.

Pulmonary fibrosis, a chronic lung condition caused by accumulation of scar tissue in the lung interstitium, can occur from many different causes; in some cases the cause is unknown. Pulmonary fibrosis presents completely different mechanical problems than emphysema: increased lung recoil, decreased lung compliance, and small lung volumes. As in emphysema, resting arterial blood gases are also variable. In mild stages of fibrosis, blood gases may be normal at rest, but in advanced stages hypercapnia and hypoxemia may prevail. (See pp. 564 and 565 in *Physiology* 3rd ed.)

CHAPTER 35

Case 1

1. *Ventilation/perfusion imbalance.* V/Q imbalance is found in virtually all forms of airway and parenchymal lung disease (asthma, pneumonia, emphysema, bronchitis, etc.). Areas of low V/Q ratios (one part of the spectrum of V/Q imbalance) cause a low PO_2 that cannot be compensated for by other areas of high V/Q ratios. In other words, low and high V/Q areas do not average out the pulmonary capillary PO_2 values, so that the final result is a lower than normal PaO_2 and a widened alveolar-arterial PO_2 difference. (See Fig. 35-3 in *Physiology* 3rd ed.)

    Using the alveolar gas equation presented in the questions for Chapter 33, we can calculate the patient's PAO_2:

$$PAO_2 = 0.21 (760 - 47) - 40 \left(0.21 + \frac{1 - 0.21}{0.8}\right) = 102 \text{ mm Hg}$$

With normal blood gases, PaO_2 would be about 90 mm Hg, and $P(A-a)O_2$ about 12 mm Hg. His $P(A-a)O_2$ is increased to 102 - 52 or 50 mm Hg, caused by pneumonia and the resulting V/Q imbalance. The V/Q imbalance in this case might also encompass some actual right to left shunting, i.e., areas of perfusion with no ventilation [V/Q = 0]).

Right to left intrapulmonary shunt. A right to left shunt can be anatomic or physiologic. An anatomic right to left shunt (e.g., a connection between a pulmonary artery and pulmonary vein that bypasses capillaries) is "fixed." Based on the clinical information (previously healthy, now acutely ill), his low PaO_2 is probably not from an anatomic shunt (which is rare in any case).

A *physiologic* right to left shunt arises from parenchymal lung disease, for example, pneumonia or pulmonary edema. Ventilation to affected areas of the lung is effectively blocked. Some perfusion continues to that area, but it does not take part in gas exchange (i.e., the blood is shunted past the unventilated alveoli). This shunted blood (with venous PO_2 and PCO_2 values) returns to the left side of the heart. As previously pointed out, a right to left intrapulmonary shunt is one extreme of V/Q imbalance (V/Q = 0).

Diffusion barrier. Diffusion block or barrier across the alveolar capillary membranes does not cause much hypoxemia in resting patients. The reason is that the reserve for oxygen transfer is quite large; normally, hemoglobin is fully loaded with oxygen after the blood has travelled about 1/3 of the way through the pulmonary capillaries. Even with a diffusion barrier, such as from fluid in the lung interstitium, oxygen usually has time to cross the alveolar-capillary membrane and fully saturate hemoglobin. The exception is if blood flow is markedly accelerated through the capillaries, as happens with strenuous exercise; then a diffusion barrier may lead to oxygen desaturation and hypoxemia.

Diseases that cause diffusion block also lead to V/Q imbalance (e.g., pulmonary edema, pneumonia), so that both physiologic abnormalities are commonly present. In such cases diffusion block is less important then V/Q imbalance in causing hypoxemia.

Hypoventilation. Hypoventilation is defined by a high $PaCO_2$, which this patient does not have; his $PaCO_2$ is low, so hypoventilation cannot be causing his hypoxemia.

In summary, the cause of his hypoxemia is V/Q imbalance, which might encompass some right to left intrapulmonary ("physiologic") shunting. (See pp. 579-589 and 594-595 in *Physiology* 3rd ed.)

2. His increased minute ventilation of 12 L/min (normally about 6 L/min at rest) with a normal Pa_{CO_2} indicates an increase in wasted ventilation. Physiologically, there are two possible causes: panting and ventilation/perfusion imbalance. Because his respiratory rate is not given, it is possible that he was breathing, for example, 50 times a minute at 200 ml/breath. Because normal anatomic dead space is about 150 ml, a tidal breath of 200 ml would give him an alveolar volume of only 50 ml/breath or an alveolar ventilation of 2.5 L (normally about 4 L/min at rest). Although hypoventilation from panting can theoretically occur without any parenchymal lung disease, it is extremely unlikely. A much more likely explanation is that V/Q imbalance has created dead space in previously normal lung tissue, by reducing perfusion more than ventilation. This is very common, particularly in patients with chronic lung diseases, such as emphysema. Because inhaled air will go to alveolar spaces whether or not they are perfused, much of each tidal volume is wasted (i.e., it goes to poorly ventilated or unventilated alveoli). Thus, V/Q imbalance causes not only hypoxemia through creation of low V/Q areas, but also wasted ventilation through creation of high V/Q areas. The latter is a principal explanation for the increased work of breathing in many patients with V/Q imbalance. They have to breathe more to bring in enough air for adequate gas exchange. (See pp. 559 and 584 in *Physiology* 3rd ed.)

3. When the patient breathes 50% oxygen, his Pa_{O_2} is only marginally better. This information does not indicate any different physiologic causes, but does implicate right to left shunting more directly as a significant feature. Without any V/Q imbalance, his Pa_{O_2} would increase by an amount predicted by the increase in F_{IO_2}. Again by the alveolar gas equation:

$$P_{AO_2} = 0.5 \ (760 - 47) - 40 \ (0.5 + \frac{1 - 0.5}{0.8}) = 317 \text{ mm Hg}$$

The variables in the equation show that P_{AO_2} is not affected by V/Q imbalance (except to the extent V/Q imbalance might affect the Pa_{CO_2}). His calculated $P(A-a)_{O_2}$ is 317 - 65 = 252 mm Hg. With normal lungs his Pa_{O_2} would be much closer to the P_{AO_2}; when he breathes 50% oxygen, P_{AO_2} should normally rise to at least 250 mm Hg. The fact that his Pa_{O_2} improved only slightly points to some degree of right to left shunting; the extra inhaled oxygen is simply not getting into his blood. We cannot reliably estimate the degree of shunt unless the subject is breathing 100% oxygen; on less than 100% oxygen, the poorly ventilated units cannot be distinguished from those not ventilated at all. (See pp. 579-581 in *Physiology* 3rd ed.)

4. When a patient breathes 100% oxygen, we can estimate the percentage of right to left shunt because all units of V/Q >0 should contain pure oxygen and should saturate the blood that perfuses them. A Pa_{O_2} lower than predicted when the patient breathes 100% oxygen reflects a right to left shunt. The percentage of shunt can be estimated as *1% of cardiac output for each 20 mm Hg P(A-a)O_2*. First, calculate P_{AO_2}.

$$P_{AO_2} = 1 \ (760 - 47) - 30 \ (1 + \frac{1 - 1}{.08}) = 673 \text{ mm Hg}$$

Next, calculate $P(A-a)_{O_2}$; in this case it is 673 - 60 = 613 mm Hg. His estimated shunt is therefore 613/20 = 31%. About 31% of his cardiac output is blood that flows through his lungs but does not

180

become oxygenated. One point to ponder: if he has such a large right to left physiologic shunt, why is his $PaCO_2$ not elevated (i.e., how is he able to exchange CO_2 so well but not O_2)? (See pp. 580, 588, and 597-598 in *Physiology* 3rd ed.)

5. The physician asks the patient to lie with his right side down. The aim is to improve perfusion to the good lung. Because his left lung is involved with pneumonia, most of his ventilation is to the right lung. Unlike ventilation, perfusion is gravity dependent. Increasing perfusion to the right lung should improve V/Q and therefore PaO_2. In fact, this change does help, and his PaO_2 increases to 77 mm Hg; intubation may therefore be avoided. (See pp. 552 and 581 in *Physiology* 3rd ed.)

6. He has a high $PaCO_2$ and therefore is hypoventilating. First use the alveolar gas equation to calculate his PAO_2.

$$PAO_2 = 0.21 (760 - 47) - 70 (0.21 + \frac{1 - 0.21}{0.8}) = 65 \text{ mm Hg}$$

Next, subtract his measured PaO_2 from the calculated PAO_2; 65 - 55 = 10 mm Hg. Because (PAO_2 - PaO_2) is normal, the cause of his low PaO_2 is simply hypoventilation (high $PaCO_2$) from the drug overdose, not a V/Q imbalance. (See pp. 559 and 588 in *Physiology* 3rd ed.)

7. The principal physiologic problem is inadequate ventilation, which is solely responsible for the hypoxemia. A comatose patient with inadequate ventilation usually requires intubation and mechanical ventilation. Giving supplemental oxygen alone, without augmenting ventilation, would transiently improve PaO_2 but not $PaCO_2$. His $PaCO_2$ could actually increase further while he receives oxygen, and lead to a fatal acidosis. (See pp. 559 and 588 in *Physiology* 3rd ed.)

Case 2

1-2. Pulmonary artery pressure and pulmonary vascular resistance will increase until the remaining lung recruits (opens up) more pulmonary capillaries, as normally occurs after a pneumonectomy. (See pp. 582-583 in *Physiology* 3rd ed.)

3-5. PaO_2 and $PaCO_2$ should remain the same because the remaining lung is handling increases in both ventilation and perfusion (i.e., V/Q ratios should not be significantly altered). (See pp. 587-588 in *Physiology* 3rd ed.)

6. For the remaining lung to accommodate twice the ventilation it normally handles, it will greatly expand its volume, even to the point of extending over to the other hemithorax. Exercise tolerance will fall because the remaining lung is stretched to its limit, and there is no or little reserve for increasing alveolar ventilation. (See pp. 607-608 in *Physiology* 3rd ed.)

CHAPTER 36

Case 1

1. The patient's HbO$_2$ equilibrium dissociation curve is shifted *downward and to the left.*

   Curve shifted down. Carbon monoxide displaces oxygen from hemoglobin at the pulmonary capillary level. This downward shift of the curve results in a lower SaO$_2$ for a given PaO$_2$. To the extent that SaO$_2$ falls, arterial oxygen content and delivery are reduced. However, the physiologic process of delivering oxygen *from* the tissue capillaries *to* the tissue cells is unaffected.

   Curve shifted to left. The curve is shifted to the left for two reasons: effect of carbon monoxide (the major reason in this example) and the increased pH (relatively minor). A left shift indicates an increase in the amount of oxygen taken up by hemoglobin in the pulmonary capillaries; this results in a higher SaO$_2$ for a given PaO$_2$. (See Fig. 36-5 and p. 594 in *Physiology* 3rd ed.) To the extent that SaO$_2$ increases, arterial oxygen content and delivery are increased. However, at the pulmonary capillary level, the leftward shift has much less effect than does the downward shift from carboxyhemoglobin; as a result, SaO$_2$ is always reduced in carbon monoxide poisoning. The leftward shift is actually detrimental, because it inhibits oxygen unloading in the systemic capillaries. Thus oxygen delivery *from* the systemic capillaries *to* the tissue cells is reduced, because hemoglobin holds on to oxygen more tightly (has increased affinity) than normal.

   In summary, excess CO adversely affects oxygenation of the patient in two ways:

   - It lowers SaO$_2$ and O$_2$ content and thereby lowers oxygen delivery *to* the systemic capillaries.

   - It impairs transport of oxygen *from* the systemic capillaries *to* the tissue cells. (See Fig. 36-5 on p. 593 in *Physiology* 3rd ed.)

2. Because this patient is breathing 100% oxygen, his PaO$_2$ amounts to about 660 mm Hg (use the alveolar gas equation provided in questions on Chapter 33). The difference between alveolar and arterial PO$_2$ normally widens with increasing FIO$_2$, but even with 100% inspired oxygen the (PAO$_2$ - PaO$_2$) should be no more than about 100 mm Hg. Hence, when the patient breathes 100% oxygen, PaO$_2$ should be at least 500 mm Hg. His PaO$_2$, while seemingly high at 190 mm Hg, is actually much less than expected for his FIO$_2$. This lower-than-expected PaO$_2$ is not caused by an excess of CO per se; CO does not affect the PaO$_2$, only the SaO$_2$ for a given PaO$_2$. The explanation for reduced PaO$_2$ must lie in V/Q imbalance, which in turn must arise from some parenchymal lung problem (e.g., pulmonary edema from smoke inhalation). Thus the physiologic data indicate a parenchymal lung problem from smoke inhalation.
   In summary, he has:

   - Excess CO, which impairs oxygen uptake by hemoglobin and oxygen delivery to the tissues,

     and

   - V/Q imbalance, not directly caused by CO, that impairs oxygen transfer across the alveolar-capillary membranes. (See pp. 588 and 594 in *Physiology* 3rd ed.)

3. CO has 250 times the affinity for hemoglobin as does oxygen. Fortunately, the binding of CO to hemoglobin is reversible; once the patient is removed from the CO source, this poison will begin to be displaced by oxygen. However, displacement is slow at physiologic P_{O_2} values (80 to 100 mm Hg), where the half-life of COHb is about 6 hours. The higher the P_{O_2}, the more quickly O_2 will displace CO from hemoglobin. Because CO-poisoned patients may die or suffer brain damage if not treated quickly, a high inspired oxygen pressure is mandatory therapy. The following table shows that the higher the Pa_{O_2}, the quicker HbCO is dissipated. (See p. 594 in *Physiology* 3rd ed.)

P_{O_2} (mm Hg)	Half-life COHb	Inspired oxygen	
100	6 hours	21%	(ambient air)
600	3 hours	100%,	at ambient air pressure
1200	2 hours	100%,	in hyperbaric chamber
1800	1 hour	100%,	in hyperbaric chamber

4. Physiologic problems rarely occur in isolation, but here you are to assume nothing else is abnormal except the indicated condition. (See pp. 559-560, 583-589, and 590-594 in *Physiology* 3rd ed.)

Condition	Pa_{O_2}	Sa_{O_2}	O_2 content
Anemia	NE	NE	D
Excess CO	NE	D	D
Fever	NE	D*	D
Acidosis	NE	D*	D
Alkalosis	NE	I*	I
Hypoventilation	D	D	D
Hyperventilation	I	I	I
V/Q imbalance	D	D	D
High altitude	D	D	D

Abbreviations: *NE*, no effect; *D*, decreased; *I*, increased.
*For a given Pa_{O_2}, effect is from shift in HbO_2 equilibrium curve.

Case 2

1. a. Arterial blood oxygen content (Ca_{O_2}) = (Sa_{O_2} x Hb x 1.34) + (0.003 x Pa_{O_2})

    b. Arterial oxygen delivery = Ca_{O_2} x cardiac output

    c. Venous blood oxygen content (Cv_{O_2}) = (Sv_{O_2} x Hb x 1.34) + (0.003 x Pv_{O_2})

    d. Oxygen uptake = (Ca_{O_2} - Cv_{O_2}) x cardiac output*

        *This important relationship is also known as the Fick Equation.

    e. Venous oxygen delivery = arterial oxygen delivery - oxygen uptake

(See pp. 556, 591, and 596 in *Physiology* 3rd ed.)

2. a.-b. Both a high $PaCO_2$ and a high temperature will shift the HbO_2 equilibrium curve to the right, thereby causing decreased oxygen uptake in the pulmonary capillaries and a reduced SaO_2. Because oxygen content is directly related to SaO_2, oxygen content will fall. Because arterial oxygen delivery is directly related to oxygen content, it too will fall. Note that the higher the PaO_2, the flatter the curve (see Fig. 36-1); compared to changes in the steep part of the curve, right and left shifts in the flat region affect pulmonary capillary oxygen uptake relatively slightly (see Fig. 36-2). The P_{50} of a right-shifted curve is higher than normal. (See pp. 590 and 592 in *Physiology* 3rd ed.)

Changes that shift the curve toward the right while causing reductions in pulmonary capillary oxygen uptake, arterial oxygen content, and arterial oxygen delivery also cause oxygen to be unloaded more easily from the venous end of the systemic capillaries, where PO_2 is low (see Fig. 36-2). Thus, although there may be less oxygen delivered to the systemic capillaries per minute, it is released to the tissues more easily; as a result, there may be no net reduction in oxygen actually delivered to the tissue cells.

   c. An increase in pH shifts the HbO_2 equilibrium curve to the left; the P_{50} will be reduced. Blood changes that shift the HbO_2 equilibrium curve toward the left lead to a higher SaO_2 at the pulmonary capillary level, although for reasons previously stated, the increase is slight in the flat portion of the curve. In this example, where pH changes from 7.5 to 7.58, SaO_2 increases only from 92% to 94%. This increase will lead to a modest increase in arterial O_2 content and delivery, which may be offset by the fact that oxygen will be held more tightly by hemoglobin at low PO_2 values (i.e., in the systemic capillaries). (See Fig. 36-2 on p. 592 in *Physiology* 3rd ed.)

   d. A 20 mm Hg increase in PaO_2 (a 33% increase over baseline) increases SaO_2 a small amount, approximately 4% (see Fig. 36-2). Because this patient's baseline pH is 7.5, the left-shifted (*solid black line*) curve in the figure more closely approximates her curve than the standard (*red line*) curve of pH 7.4. As a result of increased SaO_2, arterial oxygen content and arterial oxygen delivery will increase slightly. A change in PaO_2 by itself will not alter the position of the curve, so P_{50} will not change.

   e. Increasing hemoglobin from 9 to 12 g/dl provides a 33% increase in hemoglobin-bound oxygen content, and a corresponding increase in arterial oxygen delivery. Clearly, in the region of the flat part of the HbO_2 equilibrium curve, raising a low hemoglobin content can have a more profound effect on oxygen content and delivery than increasing PaO_2.

   f. A 20% decrease in cardiac output from 5 to 4 L/min will have no effect on oxygen content (assuming nothing else changes) but will reduce systemic oxygen delivery by the same degree, 20%. The position of the HbO_2 equilibrium curve, and hence the P_{50}, will be unaffected. (When cardiac output falls, the body usually compensates by increasing the percentage of oxygen extracted at the tissue level.) (See pp. 590-592 in *Physiology* 3rd ed.)

3. a. The percentage of oxygen taken up is the difference between arterial and venous oxygen contents divided by arterial oxygen content:

$$\frac{CaO_2 - CvO_2}{CaO_2}$$

Oxygen content = (HbO$_2$ saturation x Hb content x 1.34) + dissolved oxygen.

If you used a normal hemoglobin content of 15 g/dl blood when you did the calculation, you would find the following values (approximate):

CaO$_2$ = 20 ml O$_2$/dl
CvO$_2$ = 15 ml O$_2$/dl

In this manner the percentage of oxygen uptake is 5/20 = 25%. Note that the content can be stated as ml O$_2$/dl or ml O$_2$/L; either way the percentage of uptake is the same.

Because hemoglobin content is the same in arterial and venous blood, and dissolved oxygen is a very small amount in both arterial and venous blood, the difference in oxygen saturations also reflects the difference in contents. Normally, arterial oxygen saturation is 98% and mixed venous saturation is 75%. This difference reflects the fact that approximately 25% of arterial oxygen delivery is taken up by the tissues.

In this patient the difference in oxygen saturation (92% - 72%) indicates that about 20% of the delivered oxygen is metabolized by the tissues (i.e., about the normal amount).

b.   The percentage of total arterial oxygen delivery that returns to the right heart is 100 minus the percentage of oxygen uptake, or approximately 75%.

These values—25% oxygen uptake, 75% oxygen return to the right heart—are normal for resting individuals. The percentage of delivered oxygen used by the tissues increases in anemia, exercise, or heart failure. (See pp. 556 and 596 in *Physiology* 3rd ed.)

CHAPTER 37

Case 1

1. These blood gases are abnormal. The patient's Pa_{CO_2} is elevated, so she is hypoventilating, her pH is low as a result of the increased Pa_{CO_2}. She is also hypoxemic, with a Pa_{O_2} of 58 mm Hg; this value is explained by the increased Pa_{CO_2}. Using the alveolar gas equation, we calculate an alveolar P_{O_2} of approximately 70 mm Hg; subtracting the Pa_{O_2} results in an alveolar-arterial P_{O_2} difference of 12 mm Hg, which is within the normal range (up to 20 mm Hg). (See pp. 559 and 588 in *Physiology* 3rd ed.)

2. FVC and FEV-1 are only slightly less than the lower limit of predicted normal (80%). Also, the ratio of FEV-1 to FVC is normal and indicates no significant abnormality in air flow. Thus the patient appears to have only minimal restrictive impairment, which can be attributed to her obesity. (See p. 558 in *Physiology* 3rd ed.)

3. These spirometry values show no significant mechanical impairment. The patient has the mechanical ability to breathe and ventilate normally but lacks the drive to do so. The most likely explanation of her hypoventilation is an abnormality of the medullary brainstem that controls ventilation. Although she is certainly obese, most people with this body habitus do not hypoventilate or manifest this type of problem. (The pattern of obesity, hypoventilation, and daytime hypersomnolence is sometimes referred to as "Pickwickian syndrome," after Charles Dickens' novel *Pickwick Papers*, in which an obese character keeps falling asleep during the day.) (See p. 602 in *Physiology* 3rd ed.)

4. The features described—continued chest wall movement with absent air flow—indicate a pattern of obstructive sleep apnea. In some obese patients, the upper airway muscles don't function normally during sleep to keep the airway open, so the airway closes easily. At a critical point in airway closure the patient is aroused briefly from sleep and opens the airway (in this patient, heralded by the loud sound). Although some patients may die from the obstruction during sleep, the major problem in most patients is the recurrent hypoxemia, which can lead to pulmonary hypertension. Treatment is needed to keep her airway continually open during sleep. A variety of devices have been used to increase the air pressure during sleep and thereby keep the airway open. (See p. 606 in *Physiology* 3rd ed.)

5. The patient now manifests severe respiratory failure, pulmonary hypertension, and right-sided heart failure. Her Pa_{O_2} is lower than predicted from hypoventilation alone. The calculated Pa_{O_2} is approximately 66 mm Hg. Hence the alveolar-arterial P_{O_2} difference is 28 mm Hg. This increase indicates some ventilation-perfusion imbalance in addition to hypoventilation, and it is most likely caused by congestive heart failure. The heart failure and polycythemia are a result of chronic hypoxemia. Treatment is two-fold. Acutely, she needs mechanical ventilation. Long term, she will need to have her hypoxemia reversed, which will require continuous use of oxygen plus some device at night to prevent episodes of obstructive sleep apnea. (See p. 607 in *Physiology* 3rd ed.)

6. Her CO_2 response should be subnormal. Her history indicates that she does not increase minute ventilation appropriately when P_{CO_2} increases; a plot of her P_{CO_2} versus minute ventilation would give a line with a subnormal slope. (See p. 603 in *Physiology* 3rd ed.)

Case 2

1. It is a common misconception that F_{IO_2} falls with altitude. In fact, the F_{IO_2} is the same throughout the atmosphere (0.21).

2. Barometric pressure falls with altitude. Barometric pressure reflects the weight of the atmosphere; the less atmosphere above a certain point, the lower the barometric pressure at that point. At sea level, the barometric pressure averages 760 mm Hg. An altitude of 16,000 feet is above almost half of the earth's atmosphere, and barometric pressure is about 420 mm Hg. (The halfway point for barometric pressure, 380 mm Hg, is at about 18,000 feet altitude. On the summit of Mt. Everest, the world's highest point at 29,028 feet, barometric pressure is only 253 mm Hg.) (See p. 609 in *Physiology* 3rd ed.)

3. Pa_{O_2} falls because PA_{O_2} falls. The fall in Pa_{O_2} is predicted by the alveolar gas equation. (See p. 609 in *Physiology* 3rd ed.)

4. Pa_{CO_2} falls because hypoxic stimulation of the peripheral chemoreceptors (mainly the carotid bodies) stimulates breathing and raises the alveolar ventilation above the level of CO_2 production. Although hyperventilation effectively raises PA_{O_2} and Pa_{O_2} (approximately 1 mm Hg increase in Pa_{O_2} for every mm Hg fall in Pa_{CO_2}), the increase is not enough to overcome the fall in PA_{O_2} that results from decreased barometric pressure. Consequently, Pa_{O_2} will always fall as one ascends in altitude (assuming ambient air is breathed and one is not in a pressurized cabin). (See p. 609 in *Physiology* 3rd ed.)

5. P_{50} rises, reflecting the shift of the oxygen equilibrium curve to the right. This occurs because of a rise in 2,3-diphosphoglycerate. Although a right shift of the curve modestly decreases uptake of oxygen in the pulmonary capillaries, it unloads a greater amount of oxygen in the systemic capillaries; the net effect is enhanced oxygen transport to the tissues. (See pp. 593 and 608 in *Physiology* 3rd ed.)

6. Alveolar hypoxia constricts pulmonary arterioles and small muscular arteries, thereby increasing pulmonary vascular resistance and pulmonary artery pressure. The pressure increase would be modest and reversible on descent to sea level. (See p. 583 in *Physiology* 3rd ed.)

7. Hemoglobin content is higher in mountain dwellers, because of continued hypoxic stimulation of bone marrow by erythropoietin. (See p. 609 in *Physiology* 3rd ed.)

8. The ventilatory response to hypoxia is less than that of sea level dwellers, also because of continued exposure to low P_{O_2} conditions. (See p. 609 in *Physiology* 3rd ed.)

9. The ventilatory response to hypercapnia is unaffected by altitude. (See p. 609 in *Physiology* 3rd ed.)

10. The climber has developed acute mountain sickness, manifested by severe headache and high-altitude pulmonary edema. The cause is hypoxia, and the treatment is to increase his blood oxygen content. He should immediately receive 100% oxygen, if available. If it is not available, he must be taken to a lower altitude. This is an emergency situation and mandates immediate descent (even if he has to be carried). He might improve dramatically after descending only a few thousand feet. (See p. 610 in *Physiology* 3rd ed.)

CHAPTER 38

1. The lower part of the patient's esophagus is abnormally dilated. After subsequent swallows, the barium is mostly retained in the esophagus. In a normal individual, subsequent swallows would readily clear the barium into the stomach. (See pp. 630-632 in *Physiology* 3rd ed.)

2. The most likely explanation for the fluoroscopic observations is that the patient's LES fails to relax appropriately after a swallow. (See p. 631 in *Physiology* 3rd ed.)

3. The increased rate of emptying barium after amyl nitrate administration suggests that the patient's LES is capable of relaxing and that no structural abnormality of the LES prevents emptying of the esophagus. (See pp. 630-632 in *Physiology* 3rd ed.)

4. Esophageal manometry revealed the following abnormalities in this patient: (a) a smaller than usual increase in esophageal pressure after a swallow, (b) the failure of this pressure increase to propagate in a peristaltic fashion, (c) a higher than normal resting pressure in the LES, and (d) the failure of the LES pressure to fall as much as normal after a swallow. (See p. 631 in *Physiology* 3rd ed.)

5. The small increases in pressure that are observed after each swallow and the absence of detectable esophageal peristalsis suggest deficits of esophageal contractility and deficits in the propagation of the esophageal wave of contraction. This finding is consistent with dysfunction of the intramural plexuses of the esophagus or of the vagal motor innervation. The resting pressure in the LES is about double the normal resting LES pressure. More important, the LES fails to relax very much after a normal swallow; this might result from hypertrophy of the LES or from a deficit or malfunction in the neuronal circuitry that mediates LES relaxation. In the normal individual, the LES relaxes essentially completely after a swallow to allow esophageal propulsion to proceed. This dysfunction of the LES is the major problem in the patient's disorder, which is known as *achalasia*. (See p. 631 in *Physiology* 3rd ed.)

6. Because the esophageal sphincter remains closed, when the upper part of the esophagus (which appears to be close to normal in this disorder) contracts, the pressure is transmitted down the esophagus with essentially no time delay, because water is incompressible. (See p. 631 in *Physiology* 3rd ed.)

7. Forceful dilation of the LES tears some of the esophageal muscle fibers. This makes it possible for the LES to relax sufficiently after a swallow to allow swallowing to be almost normal. (See pp. 630-633 in *Physiology* 3rd ed.)

8. With time the damage done to the LES is repaired, and the original problems with swallowing, caused by failure of the LES to relax sufficiently, recur. (See p. 633 in *Physiology* 3rd ed.)

9. The therapeutic options at this point are the same as those available when the disorder was first diagnosed: (a) to treat the patient with drugs (calcium channel blockers such as nifedipine taken by mouth just before eating), (b) to repeat the abrupt mechanical dilation of the LES, (c) to make a longitudinal incision in the LES through the entire thickness of the musculature, which markedly weakens the LES. (See pp. 381 and 633 in *Physiology* 3rd ed.)

CHAPTER 39

1. The dramatically elevated serum gastrin level in the patient might be responsible for the elevated rate of HCl secretion. The increased density of gastric glands and increased population of parietal cells within the glands in the biopsy specimen might also contribute to elevated HCl secretion. (See pp. 665-668 in *Physiology* 3rd ed.)

2. Because HCl itself promotes the release of pepsinogen, the secretion of pepsinogen by the patient is expected to be somewhat elevated. This should contribute to the ulceration of the patient's duodenum. (See p. 669 in *Physiology* 3rd ed.)

3. The patient's stomach secretes HCl at rates far above normal. The amount of HCl that enters the duodenum is probably too great to be neutralized there by pancreatic, biliary, and duodenal secretions, and thereby causes the pH in the duodenum to be much lower than normal. In addition to the low pH, the elevated levels of pepsins may contribute to the damage of the duodenal mucosa. (See pp. 660 and 669 in *Physiology* 3rd ed.)

4. Gastric ulcers are rarely associated with hypersecretion of HCl. The gastric mucosal barrier (mucus and bicarbonate) normally suffices to protect the stomach even in hypersecretors. Gastric ulcers are usually the result of a defect in the gastric mucosal barrier. For this reason, patients with gastric ulcers are usually hyposecretors of HCl; this is because of the strong inhibitory effect of the low pH at the surface of the antral mucosa on secretion of HCl. (See pp. 663 and 664 in *Physiology* 3rd ed.)

5. There are several causes of high serum gastrin. Patients who are *hypo*secretors of gastric acid for any reason (such as pernicious anemia or achlorhydria) have elevated serum gastrin, because the negative feedback induced by low pH in the antrum is a major brake on gastrin secretion by antral G cells. This patient is a hypersecretor of HCl, so those causes can be ruled out. The most prominent possibilities that remain are hyperplasia of antral G cells or the presence (not in the stomach) of a gastrinoma (a gastrin-secreting tumor). Gastrinomas occur most frequently in the pancreas and are the cause of the disorder known as *Zollinger-Ellison syndrome*. (See pp. 664-668 and 709 in *Physiology* 3rd ed.)

6. Pancreatic lipase is extremely pH sensitive and can be rapidly and irreversibly denatured at acid pH. The inactivation of lipase because of the low duodenal pH in this patient is the most likely cause of her steatorrhea. (See pp. 710 and 714 in *Physiology* 3rd ed.)

7. The patient's steatorrhea probably contributes to the diarrhea. Certain fatty acids are hydroxylated by intestinal bacteria to form compounds that induce secretion of fluid and electrolytes by colonic epithelial cells. In addition, gastrin at high levels induces secretion and inhibits absorption of fluid and electrolytes in the small intestine. (See pp. 703 and 714 in *Physiology* 3rd ed.)

8. Gastrin has a trophic effect on the oxyntic mucosa. The constant high level of serum gastrin in this patient is probably responsible for the increased number of gastric glands in the fundus and the increased density of parietal cells in the glands of the fundus. (See p. 666 in *Physiology* 3rd ed.)

9. After a meal, peptides and amino acids in the stomach and gastric distension stimulate antral and jejunal G cells to release gastrin. If the patient's high serum gastrin were caused by hyperplasia of antral or jejunal G cells, a significant rise in gastrin after a meal would be expected. If, on the other hand, the high serum gastrin is caused by a gastrinoma (Zollinger-Ellison syndrome), no significant

rise in gastrin is expected after a meal. This finding suggests that the patient has Zollinger-Ellison syndrome. (See p. 667 in *Physiology* 3rd ed.)

10. Secretin strongly suppresses gastric HCl secretion, primarily by a direct inhibition of the parietal cells. In a normal individual, secretin has little effect on the secretion of gastrin. By mechanisms that have not been fully elucidated, secretin stimulates gastrinoma cells to release gastrin. This finding pretty well clinches the diagnosis of Zollinger-Ellison syndrome. (See p. 668 in *Physiology* 3rd ed.)

11. Gastrin is a relatively weak secretagogue at the parietal cell. Gastrin mostly effects HCl secretion by releasing histamine from ECL cells in the gastric mucosa. Hence, cimetidine, which blocks the histamine H_2 receptors on the parietal cells, blocks much of the effect of the elevated serum gastrin in this patient. The binding of cimetidine to H_2 receptors is reversible. Moreover, cimetidine is degraded and excreted at a fairly high rate. For this reason, and because of the very high gastrin levels in this patient, large and frequent doses of cimetidine are required to suppress HCl secretion sufficiently to allow the patient's ulcer to heal. (See p. 666 in *Physiology* 3rd ed.)

12. Acetylcholine is a secretagogue at the parietal cell and also elicits secretion of histamine by gastric ECL cells. There is a potentiation between gastrin and acetylcholine at both cell types. Suppression of cholinergic drive with an anticholinergic drug lessens the effectiveness of the elevated gastrin at the levels of the parietal cell and the ECL cell. In this way, the anticholinergic drug enhances the effectiveness of cimetidine in this patient. (See pp. 664-666 in *Physiology* 3rd ed.)

13. Omeprazole inhibits the H^+, K^+-ATPase in parietal cells. It is thus a potent inhibitor of gastric acid secretion evoked by any secretagogue. Omeprazole forms a covalent bond with the H^+, K^+-ATPase and inhibits it irreversibly. The inhibition is only relieved by the synthesis of new H^+, K^+-ATPase molecules. For this reason, the inhibition of HCl secretion by omeprazole in this patient is longer lasting than that by other drugs. (See p. 661 in *Physiology* 3rd ed.)

14. The first priority is to locate the gastrinoma(s) in this patient with Zollinger-Ellison syndrome. If gastrinomas can be identified, they should be removed. Because over half of the gastrinomas in Zollinger-Ellison patients are malignant, chemotherapy may be appropriate. Zollinger-Ellison patients often become refractory to treatment with H_2 receptor antagonists. Other treatments that may be used include proximal vagotomy (sectioning the vagal branches to the fundus and the body of the stomach) and partial or total gastrectomy. Omeprazole has been available only recently and it is too early to determine whether omeprazole therapy will supplant vagotomy and gastrectomy in the long-term management of Zollinger-Ellison patients. (See pp. 661 and 666 in *Physiology* 3rd ed.)

CHAPTER 40

1. The brush border plasma membranes of the proximal renal tubule and the jejunum contain similar transport proteins that couple the downhill transport of Na^+ ions into the cells with the active transport of amino acids into the cell. The amino acids present at high concentrations in the patient's urine are primarily those that are transported by the neutral brush border (NBB) amino acid transport system. These data are explained by a defect in the NBB transporter in the proximal tubule brush border plasma membrane. Thus, most filtered neutral amino acids cannot be reabsorbed quantitatively by the proximal tubule, in contrast to normal individuals. (See pp. 695-697 in *Physiology* 3rd ed.)

2. This observation is consistent with the explanation that the same NBB amino acid transporter that is deficient in the renal proximal tubule is also deficient in the jejunal brush border. Thus the ability to absorb these neutral amino acids as free amino acids from the intestinal lumen is diminished. (See pp. 695-697 in *Physiology* 3rd ed.)

3. Dipeptides and tripeptides are absorbed avidly in the jejunum by a peptide transporter. Oligopeptides fed to the patient are reduced to dipeptides and tripeptides by the combined action of pepsins, pancreatic proteases, and brush border peptidases. The various individual neutral amino acids are then absorbed in the form of mixed dipeptides and tripeptides. (See p. 695 in *Physiology* 3rd ed.)

4. A fraction of a normal individual's niacin (nicotinamide) is provided by its synthesis from tryptophan. The major pathway for degradation of tryptophan ends in the production of nicotinamide. Because the patient cannot reabsorb tryptophan from his urine, levels of this amino acid fall and, as a result, less conversion of tryptophan to nicotinamide occurs. This problem may be exacerbated because the degradation of 60 mg of tryptophan is required to produce 1 mg of nicotinamide. Thus the diminished availability of tryptophan causes the patient to be deficient in niacin, despite having an amount of niacin in his diet that would be adequate for a normal individual. (See p. 708 in *Physiology* 3rd ed.)

5. Patients with this disorder (as judged from high concentrations of neutral amino acids in urine) are much more likely to have symptoms if they also have poor diets. A patient with a high-protein diet is believed to compensate somewhat for the loss of tryptophan by increasing absorption of tryptophan (from dipeptides and tripeptides) in the jejunum. A patient with a high intake of niacin is also less likely to be symptomatic. (See p. 695 in *Physiology* 3rd ed.)

6. The patient is not malnourished, because sufficient amounts of those neutral amino acids that are transported by the NBB system can be absorbed in the jejunum as dipeptides and tripeptides to supply the requirement of protein synthesis for the essential amino acids. (See p. 695 in *Physiology* 3rd ed.)

7. Pellagra is the disease that results from dietary deficiency of niacin. There is no deficiency in the conversion of tryptophan to niacin in pellagra. This patient has Hartnup syndrome in which the deficiency is in the renal and intestinal transport of tryptophan, which diminishes the conversion of tryptophan to nicotinamide. (See pp. 696, 697, and 708 in *Physiology* 3rd ed.)

CHAPTER 41

Case 1

A. Because of the damage to the capillary endothelium and basement membrane, red blood cells would be found in the urine; this is termed *hematuria*. Importantly, red blood cells can also appear in the urine even when the filtration barrier is not damaged. For example, red blood cells can appear in the urine as a result of bleeding in any part of the lower urinary tract. Such bleeding occurs with kidney stones, and occasionally as a result of a bacterial infection that occurs in the lower urinary tract and causes bleeding. In women, urine can also contain menstrual blood.

B. Because glucose is filtered and completely reabsorbed by the proximal tubule, it is not normally found in the urine. Its presence in the urine indicates either (a) an elevated plasma glucose level, such that the filtered load (i.e., GFR x P glucose) is greater than the T_m for glucose reabsorption by the proximal tubule, or (b) an abnormality in glucose transport. Because glucose is freely filtered by the normal glomerulus, damage to the ultrafiltration barrier would not increase its filtration.

C. Na^+ normally appears in the urine of healthy individuals. Like glucose, Na^+ is freely filtered by the normal glomerulus. Therefore damage to the filtration barrier does not increase the rate of Na^+ excretion.

D. Normally the urine contains essentially no protein because the glomerulus prevents the filtration of plasma proteins. However, when the glomerulus is damaged, large amounts of plasma proteins can be filtered. If the amount filtered overwhelms the reabsorptive capacity of the proximal tubule, protein appears in the urine (proteinuria). (See p. 734 in *Physiology* 3rd ed.)

Case 2

This problem makes use of the relationship:

Excretion rate = filtered load - excretion rate + secretion rate

$$U_x \cdot \dot{V} = (GFR \cdot P_x) - R + S$$

Insulin: the clearance of inulin provides a measure of the GFR:

$$GFR = \frac{U_x \cdot \dot{V}}{P_x}$$

Substance	Urine [x] (mg/ml)	Plasma [x] (mg/ml)	$U_x \cdot V$ (mg/min)	Clearance (ml/min)	Filtered load (mg/min)	Transport rate (mg/min)
Inulin	5.5	0.025	2.75	110.0	2.75	0
A	0.8	0.040	0.40	10.0	4.40	4.0 Reab.
B	7.5	0.068	3.75	55.1	3.74	≈ 0
C	11.0	0.010	5.50	550.0	1.10	4.4 Secrt.
D	10.0	0.060	5.0	83.3	1.65	3.4 Secrt.

A.   This substance is freely filtered and almost entirely reabsorbed.

B.   This substance is 50% bound to plasma protein. The total plasma [x] is used to calculate clearance, but only the free [x] is used to calculate the filtered load. Because the filtered load equals the excretion rate, there is no tubular transport.

C.   This substance is freely filtered and also secreted.

D.   This substance is 75% bound to plasma protein. Because the filtered load is less than the excretion rate, the substance is secreted. Note: if it were not known that substances B and D were bound to plasma protein, examination of their clearances would have led to the erroneous conclusion that both were reabsorbed by the nephron. (See p. 733 in *Physiology* 3rd ed.)

Case 3

Urination (micturition) occurs as a result of a spinal cord reflex involving sympathetic and parasympathetic fibers. The fibers and spinal cord interneurons involved in this reflex exit the spinal cord below the first lumbar vertebra. The motor and sensory deficits in this patient would suggest a lesion above this level. Consequently, it would be expected that the micturition reflex would be intact. Thus, filling of the bladder with urine would trigger the reflex and would result in micturition. However, the loss of input from higher centers in the CNS would not allow the man to control this reflex. He would have no sensation of a full bladder and would not be able to inhibit the reflex. In many ways micturition in this man would resemble that of a newborn baby. Because the skeletal muscles that comprise the external sphincter are under voluntary control, leakage of urine (incontinence) will also occur. (See pp. 725-727 in *Physiology* 3rd ed.)

CHAPTER 42

Case 1

The initial volumes of the body fluid compartments and the osmoles in these compartments are calculated as follows (osmolality is estimated as 2 x [Na$^+$]):

Initial total body water	= 0.6 x (60 kg) = 36 L
Initial ICF volume	= 0.4 x (60 kg) = 24 L
Initial ECF volume	= 0.2 x (60 kg) = 12 L
Initial total body osmoles	= (total body water) (body fluid osmolality)
	=(36 L)(280 mOsm/kg H$_2$O) = 10,080 mOsm
Initial ICF osmoles	= (ICF volume)(body fluid osmolality)
	=(24 L)(280 mOsm/kg H$_2$O) = 6720 mOsm
Initial ECF osmoles	= total body osmoles - ICF osmoles
	=10,080 mOsm - 6720 mOsm = 3360 mOsm

4 kg of body weight is lost. It is assumed that this entire weight reduction reflects fluids lost through vomiting and diarrhea. Thus, 4 L of fluid is lost. Because the plasma [Na$^+$] is unchanged, a proportional amount of solute was also lost (isotonic loss of fluid). There will be no fluid shifts between the ECF and ICF, because of the absence of an osmotic gradient between these compartments. Thus the ECF loses 4 L of volume and 4 x 280 = 1120 mOsm of solute.

New total body water	= 36 L - 4 L = 32 L
New ICF volume	= 24 L (unchanged)
New ECF volume	= 12 L - 4 L = 8 L
New total body osmoles	= 10,080 mOsm - 1120 mOsm = 8960 mOsm
New ICF osmoles	= 6720 mOsm (unchanged)
New ECF osmoles	= 3360 mOsm - 1120 mOsm = 2240 mOsm

(See pp. 756-758 in *Physiology* 3rd ed.)

Case 2

The initial volumes of the body fluid compartments and the osmoles in these compartments are calculated as for problem I:

Initial total body water	= 0.6 x (50 kg) = 30 L
Initial ICF volume	= 0.4 x (50 kg) = 20 L
Initial ECF volume	= 0.2 x (50 kg) = 10 L
Initial total body osmoles	= (total body water)(body fluid osmolality)
	= (30 L)(290 mOsm/kg H$_2$O) = 8700 mOsm
Initial ICF osmoles	= (ICF volume)(body fluid osmolality)
	= (20 L)(290 mOsm/kg H$_2$O) = 5800 mOsm
Initial ECF osmoles	= total body osmoles - ICF osmoles
	= 8700 mOsm - 5800 mOsm = 2900 mOsm

To determine the effect of the mannitol, the total amount infused must first be calculated. At 5 g/kg, a total of 250 g was infused (1.374 moles of mannitol). Because mannitol is a single particle in solution, this adds

1,374 mOsm to the ECF. The mannitol will raise ECF osmolality and result in the shift of fluid from the ICF into the ECF.

New total body water	= 30 L (unchanged)
New total body osmoles	= 8700 mOsm + 1374 mOsm = 10,074 mOsm
New ICF osmoles	= 5800 mOsm (unchanged)
New ECF osmoles	= 2900 mOsm + 1374 mOsm = 4274 mOsm

$$\text{New plasma osmolality} = \frac{\text{new total osmoles}}{\text{total body water}}$$

$$\frac{10,074 \text{ mOsm}}{30 \text{ L}} = 336 \text{ mOsm/kg H}_2\text{O}$$

$$\text{New ICF volume} = \frac{\text{ICF osmoles}}{\text{New P}_{osm}} = \frac{5800 \text{ mOsm}}{336 \text{ mOsm/kg H}_2\text{O}} = 17.3 \text{ L}$$

New ECF volume = total body water - ICF volume
= 30 L - 17.3 = 12.7 L

Because mannitol increases the osmolality of the ECF, 2.7 L of fluid shifts from the ICF into the ECF. To calculate the new plasma $[Na^+]$, it is assumed that the amount of Na^+ in the ECF is unchanged after mannitol infusion. Originally, there were 2900 mOsm attributed to Na^+ (2 x $[Na^+]$ x ECF volume) in the ECF. Because the Na^+ osmoles are unchanged but now present in a larger volume, the new plasma $[Na^+]$ is calculated as follows:

$$\text{New plasma Na}^+ \text{ osmoles} = \frac{2900 \text{ mOsm due to Na}^+}{12.7\text{L}} = 228 \text{ mOsm/L}$$

$$\text{New plasma } [Na^+] = \frac{\text{Na}^+ \text{ osmoles}}{2} = \frac{228 \text{ mOsm}}{2} = 114 \text{ mEq/L}$$

(See pp. 756-758 in *Physiology* 3rd ed.)

Case 3

This problem illustrates the importance of effective versus ineffective osmoles in regulating ADH secretion. Although plasma osmolality is elevated, the increased osmolality is caused by urea. Because urea is an ineffective osmole with regard to ADH secretion, it is necessary to estimate the osmolality of plasma that is caused by effective osmoles (Na^+ and its anions). The effective osmolality of the plasma is estimated by doubling the plasma $[Na^+]$, which yields a value of 270 mOsm/kg H_2O. Because the effective osmolality is reduced from normal (normal is 280 to 290 mOsm/kg H_2O), ADH secretion is suppressed and plasma levels are reduced. (See pp. 758-760 in *Physiology* 3rd ed.)

Case 4

It is assumed that the 3 kg weight loss reflects only the loss of fluid. Because the plasma [Na^+] is unchanged, this represents a loss of isotonic fluid (3 L) from the ECF.

Plasma osmolality: because the plasma [Na^+] is unchanged, the plasma osmolality is unchanged.

Effective circulating volume (ECV): the loss of fluid from the ECF will decrease the effective circulating volume.

ADH secretion: the decrease in ECV, through the vascular baroreceptors, will stimulate ADH secretion.

Urine osmolality: the increased levels of ADH will lead to water conservation by the kidneys, and a concentrated urine will be excreted.

Sensation of thirst: again, the decrease in ECV, through the vascular baroreceptors, will lead to an enhanced sensation of thirst.

(See pp. 770-775 and 779-780 in *Physiology* 3rd ed.)

Case 5

The woman is euvolemic. To maintain Na^+ balance, the amount of Na^+ ingested in the diet must equal the amount excreted from the body. Because the kidneys are the primary route for Na^+ excretion, the amount of Na^+ excreted daily is nearly equal to the amount ingested in the diet (small amounts of Na^+ are lost in perspiration and feces). Therefore the Na^+ excretion rate in this woman is approximately 200 mEq/day. (See pp. 770-775 and 779-780 in *Physiology* 3rd ed.)

Case 6

This man has gained 4 kg. This represents the accumulation of 4 L of fluid (1 kg = 1 L) in the ECF. A portion of the fluid will accumulate in the interstitial fluid compartments as edema. The composition of this fluid is the same as that of plasma and has a [Na^+] of 145 mEq/L. Recall that the accumulation of the fluid requires Na^+ retention by the kidneys. Therefore the amount of Na^+ retained by the kidneys must be equal to the amount contained in 4 L of fluid having a [Na^+] of 145 mEq/L, or 580 mEq of Na^+. (See pp. 775, 781, and 782 in *Physiology* 3rd ed.)

Case 7

Aldosterone stimulates Na^+ reabsorption in the collecting duct, which explains the reduction in Na^+ secretion seen initially. As a result of the positive Na^+ balance, the effective circulating blood volume is increased. This in turn reduces proximal tubule reabsorption and enhances delivery of Na^+ to the collecting duct. Additionally, atrial natriuretic peptide (ANP) levels are increased, and its action on the collecting duct to inhibit Na^+ reabsorption, together with increased Na^+ delivery, returns the Na^+ excretion to its previous level. A new steady state is reached in which ECV is expanded, and hence the body weight is increased. With removal of the adenoma and return of the aldosterone levels to normal, the Na^+ reabsorptive rate of the collecting duct decreases. Because of the increased ECV and therefore enhanced Na^+ delivery to the collecting duct, the reabsorptive capacity of the collecting duct is overwhelmed, and Na^+ excretion increases. After a period of negative Na^+ balance, the ECV decreases back to normal. A new steady state is reached, and the body weight returns to its original value as the extracellular fluid volume decreases. (See pp. 772-775 and 777-778 in *Physiology* 3rd ed.)

Case 8

1. The ECF volume of this man is increased above normal. The presence of edema, distension of the neck veins, and rales (sounds caused by fluid) in the lungs are evidence of this increased volume. Additional evidence could be obtained by measuring weight gain, because accumulation of each liter of extracellular fluid would increase body weight by 1 kg. (See pp. 780-782 in *Physiology* 3rd ed.)

2. The ECV in this man would be decreased below normal. With damage to the myocardium, cardiac output and therefore tissue perfusion would be reduced; this would be sensed by the body as a decrease in the ECV. The ECV cannot be measured directly. Therefore to determine if the ECV is reduced, measurements would have to be made of parameters that change in response to alterations in the ECV. For example, the kidneys reduce Na^+ excretion in response to a decrease in the ECV. Measurement of fractional Na^+ excretion could confirm the existence of a reduced effective circulating volume (fraction Na^+ excretion < 1%). However, in this man fractional excretion may not be very low because a thiazide diuretic was used. Alternatively, measurements would be made of plasma renin activity because this would be stimulated by the decreased ECV. (See pp. 771 and 779-780 in *Physiology* 3rd ed.)

3. The kidneys would be avidly retaining Na^+. With a decrease in the effective circulating volume, sensors in the low-pressure (cardiac atria and pulmonary vasculature) and high-pressure (juxtaglomerular apparatus, aortic arch, and carotid sinus) sides of the circulation would be activated, and the signals would be sent to the kidneys to retain Na^+.

    *   Sympathetic nerves that innervate the afferent and efferent arterioles of the glomeruli would cause vasoconstriction. The net result would be to reduce the GFR; this in turn would reduce the filtered load of Na^+.

    *   Sympathetic innervation of the proximal tubule and the thick ascending limb of Henle's loop will also increase Na^+ reabsorption at these sites.

    *   Increased sympathetic nerve activity, together with decreased perfusion pressure at the afferent arteriole, will result in the secretion of renin. This activation of the renin-angiotensin-aldosterone system will further stimulate Na^+ reabsorption, because angiotensin II stimulates proximal tubule Na^+ reabsorption, and aldosterone stimulates Na^+ reabsorption in the distal tubule and collecting duct. With the increase in the ECV, atrial natriuretic peptide (ANP) levels will be elevated. However, the effect of ANP (inhibition of renin secretion and natriuresis) appears to be blunted by the effect of the other factors, all of which act to reduce Na^+ excretion.

    The net effect of these responses is retention of Na^+ by the kidneys. As a result of this Na^+ retention (positive Na^+ balance), the ECF volume will increase and lead to the formation of edema, as seen in the physical examination of this man. (See pp. 739, 772-775, and 779-782 in *Physiology* 3rd ed.)

4. The development of hyponatremia indicates that this man is in positive water balance. In this case the ingestion of water has exceeded the capacity of the kidneys to excrete solute-free water. Solute-free water excretion is impaired in this man for several reasons:

- ADH secretion is stimulated because of the decreased ECV. As a consequence, solute-free water is reabsorbed by the collecting duct.

- The filtered load of solute (NaCl) and water is reduced, and fractional reabsorption by the proximal tubule is enhanced. As a result, delivery of solute and water to the thick ascending limb (the primary site where solute-free water is generated) is decreased.

- The thiazide diuretic inhibits NaCl reabsorption in the distal tubule. This portion of the nephron also participates in the generation of solute-free water. With impaired NaCl reabsorption less solute-free water can be generated. (See pp. 760 and 768-770 in *Physiology* 3rd ed.)

5. Hypokalemia in this man is the result of increased renal K^+ excretion. Two factors contribute to stimulating K^+ excretion. The first is related to the administration of the thiazide diuretic. Thiazide diuretics act on the early portion of the distal tubule to inhibit NaCl reabsorption. Inhibition of NaCl reabsorption in the distal tubule results in the delivery of increased quantities of Na^+ and fluid to the portion of the nephron responsible for K^+ secretion (cortical portion of the collecting duct). This increased delivery stimulates K^+ secretion by the principal cells in this part of the nephron. Second, the ECV is decreased in this man, which in turn stimulates the renin-angiotensin-aldosterone system. Aldosterone then acts on the collecting duct to stimulate K^+ secretion. The enhanced secretion of K^+ by the collecting duct will result in increased K^+ excretion and the development of hypokalemia. Extrarenal factors will also contribute to the development of hypokalemia because both alkalosis and aldosterone cause K^+ to move into cells. (See pp. 784-786, 788, and 789 in *Physiology* 3rd ed.)

6. Although an arterial blood sample was not obtained, the plasma $[HCO_3]$ is elevated, suggesting the presence of a metabolic alkalosis. The development of a metabolic alkalosis could reflect enhanced renal HCO_3 reabsorption and H^+ excretion. HCO_3 reabsorption by the proximal tubule would be stimulated because proximal tubule reabsorption is enhanced when the ECV is decreased (see the answer to question 3). Virtually all of the filtered load of HCO_3 will be reabsorbed by the time the tubular fluid reaches the distal tubule and collecting duct. H^+ secretion at these sites will titrate urinary buffers and lead to the generation of "new HCO_3." Because of the decreased ECV, aldosterone levels are elevated. Because aldosterone stimulates H^+ secretion in the distal tubule and collecting duct, "new HCO_3" generation will be increased, and metabolic alkalosis will develop. (See pp. 799-804 in *Physiology* 3rd ed.)

7. Creatinine is excreted from the body mainly by glomerular filtration (10% is excreted as a result of secretion by the proximal tubule). Therefore the amount of creatinine excreted is determined mainly by its filtered load. With a reduction in the ECV, the glomerular filtration rate is reduced (see the answer to question 3). The reduced filtration rate will decrease the filtered load of creatinine, and thus its excretion. As a result, the serum [creatinine] will increase. The serum [creatinine] should return to normal when the ECV is restored to its normal value. (See pp. 728 and 729 in *Physiology* 3rd ed.)

8. A loop diuretic will act on the thick ascending limb of Henle's loop to inhibit NaCl reabsorption and increase Na^+ excretion. This enhanced excretion of Na^+ will further decrease the ECV. The loop diuretic can further reduce the serum Na^+ and K^+ concentrations, make the metabolic alkalosis worse, and further increase the serum [creatinine].

- The thick ascending limb of Henle's loop is the primary site where tubular fluid is diluted. The loop diuretic will inhibit the separation of solute (NaCl) and water at this site and further impair the generation of solute-free water (see the answer to question 4). If water ingestion is not reduced, hyponatremia could become more severe. (See pp. 760 and 768-770 in *Physiology* 3rd ed.)

- The thick ascending limb of Henle's loop reabsorbs approximately 20% of the filtered load of K^+. This process is inhibited by loop diuretics. Also, the loop diuretic will cause increased delivery of Na^+ and fluid to the K^+ secretory site. Together, these effects will further enhance K^+ secretion and thus renal K^+ excretion, leading to a worsening of the hypokalemia. (See pp. 788 and 789 in *Physiology* 3rd ed.)

- Because the loop diuretic leads to a further reduction in the ECV, the stimuli for enhancing both proximal tubule HCO_3 reabsorption and distal tubule and collecting duct H^+ secretion will be increased. As a result, the metabolic alkalosis may become more severe. (See pp. 799-804 in *Physiology* 3rd ed.)

- With the added decrement in the ECV caused by the loop diuretic, the glomerular filtration rate will fall further and thereby cause the serum [creatinine] to increase. (See pp. 728 and 729 in *Physiology* 3rd ed.)

The abnormalities in serum electrolytes seen in this man are caused mainly by the decreased ECV, which was a result of his myocardial infarction. The diuretic therapy is directed at preventing the kidneys from responding to the decreased ECV. Although the diuretics reduce Na^+ retention by the kidneys and help alleviate edema formation, they decrease further the ECV and thus may produce the water, Na^+, K^+ and acid-base abnormalities seen in this patient.

CHAPTER 43

Case 1

pH	[HCO$_3^-$] (mEq/L)	P$_{CO_2}$ (mm Hg)	Disorder
7.34	15	29	Metabolic acidosis
7.49	35	48	Metabolic alkalosis
7.47	14	20	Chronic respiratory alkalosis
7.34	31	60	Chronic respiratory acidosis
7.26	26	60	Acute respiratory acidosis
7.62	20	20	Acute respiratory alkalosis
7.09	15	50	Metabolic + respiratory acidosis
7.40	15	25	Metabolic acidosis + respiratory alkalosis

The first six disorders are simple acid-base disorders. Mixed metabolic and respiratory acidosis is seen during cardiopulmonary arrest. With cessation of cardiac function, the tissues are inadequately perfused and resort to anaerobic metabolism (production of lactic acid). With cessation of respiration, CO_2 is retained. In the example of mixed metabolic acidosis and respiratory alkalosis, pH is normal, but both the [HCO$_3^-$] and P$_{CO_2}$ are abnormal. An example of a clinical condition that produces such a disorder is an overdose of aspirin. The metabolic acidosis is the result of the salicylic acid (active ingredient of aspirin), and the respiratory alkalosis is the result of hyperventilation secondary to salicylic acid stimulation of the respiratory centers. (See p. 807 in *Physiology* 3rd ed.)

Case 2

The initial set of laboratory data indicates the presence of a metabolic alkalosis with appropriate respiratory compensation. Given the man's history, the most likely cause of this simple acid-base disorder is the loss of gastric acid by vomiting. The second set of laboratory data continues to show the presence of a metabolic alkalosis with respiratory compensation. In addition, fluid loss is evident (decrease in body weight by 2 kg) and, as a result, a contracted ECV (decrease in blood pressure). Given the worsening of this man's metabolic alkalosis, it is somewhat surprising that the urine pH is so acidic. The appropriate renal response should be an increase in HCO$_3^-$ excretion to correct the alkalosis. However, by decreasing the filtered load of HCO$_3^-$ (decreased GFR) and stimulating proximal Na$^+$ reabsorption, the decreased ECV prevents the excretion of HCO$_3^-$ (HCO$_3^-$ reabsorption is linked to Na$^+$). To correct this situation, the ECV must be restored to its normal value. Infusion of isotonic NaCl would accomplish this and also allow the kidneys to excrete the excess HCO$_3^-$, and thereby restores acid-base balance. (See pp. 799-802 in *Physiology* 3rd ed.)

Case 3
Carbonic anhydrase plays a critical role in the reabsorption of HCO$_3^-$ by the cells of the proximal tubule and by intercalated cells of the collecting duct. Inhibition of this enzyme would therefore inhibit the reabsorption of HCO$_3^-$ at these nephron sites. Because of the large fraction of the filtered load of HCO$_3^-$ reabsorbed by the proximal tubule, the effect at this site is quantitatively more important. With decreased reabsorption, more HCO$_3^-$ would be excreted in the urine, and urine pH would become alkaline. This loss of HCO$_3^-$ from the body would result in the development of a metabolic acidosis. (See pp. 799-801 in *Physiology* 3rd ed.)

Case 4

Intravenous infusion of K^+ into a subject with a combination of sympathetic blockade and insulin deficiency would result in greater hyperkalemia than would a similar infusion of K^+ in a normal subject. Although aldosterone secretion would be stimulated by the hyperkalemia, this hormone stimulates cell K^+ uptake after a one-hour lag period. In this first hour after K^+ infusion, less than 50% of the infused K^+ is excreted by the kidneys. Because sympathetic activity and insulin release are suppressed, most of the K^+ in the body will remain in the extracellular fluid. (See pp. 784 and 785 in *Physiology* 3rd ed.)

Case 5

1. The symptoms and the electrolyte disturbances of this woman are most characteristic of decreased levels of adrenal cortical steroids, and especially the mineralocorticoid hormone aldosterone. This patient has Addison's disease. The presence of hyperpigmentation suggests that the problem is at the level of the adrenal gland. ACTH levels are elevated in response to the decreased circulating levels of adrenal cortical steroids. These elevated levels of ACTH stimulate melanocytes and cause hyperpigmentation. (See p. 970 in *Physiology* 3rd ed.)

2. The hypotension is a result of the negative Na^+ balance present in this woman,, which in turn reflects the decreased circulating levels of aldosterone. With hypoaldosteronism, Na^+ reabsorption by the collecting duct is reduced, and negative Na^+ balance develops (Na^+ excretion > Na^+ intake). Because ECF volume reflects Na^+ balance, ECF volume will be decreased. Because plasma is a component of the ECF, vascular volume and hence blood pressure will be decreased. (See pp. 756-762 and 770-771 in *Physiology* 3rd ed.)

3. Hyponatremia indicates a problem in water metabolism. Thus the ability of this woman's kidneys to excrete solute-free water is impaired, and she is in positive water balance (solute-free water ingestion > solute-free water excretion). Excretion of solute-free water is impaired for two primary reasons, both of which are related to decreased effective circulating blood volume. With the decreased effective circulating blood volume, the glomerular filtration rate is reduced, which reduces the filtered load of solute (NaCl) and water. Also, the proximal tubules reabsorb a greater fraction of the filtered load of NaCl. Together, these effects reduce the delivery of solute and water to the thick ascending limb of Henle's loop; i.e., the portion of the nephron where solute-free water is generated. In addition, the decreased effective circulating volume causes the secretion of ADH. With ADH present, the collecting duct will reabsorb water and thereby reduce its excretion. (See pp. 770 and 779-780 in *Physiology* 3rd ed.)

4. Urinary K^+ excretion is determined mostly by the amount of K^+ secreted into tubular fluid by the distal tubule and collecting duct. K^+ secretion at these nephron sites is reduced by a decrease in the serum [aldosterone], as well as in the [Na^+] and flow rate of the tubular fluid. Therefore, K^+ excretion by the distal tubule and collecting duct will be reduced in this woman, and she will be in positive K^+ balance (intake > excretion). In addition, aldosterone causes the uptake of K^+ into cells (e.g., skeletal muscle). In the absence of aldosterone, cellular uptake will be less. This will contribute to the development of hyperkalemia. (See pp. 784-788 in *Physiology* 3rd ed.)

5. This woman's acid-base disturbance is likely to be metabolic acidosis secondary to reduced net acid excretion by the kidneys. Although arterial blood pH is not reported, the reduced plasma [HCO_3^-] is consistent with a metabolic acidosis. Net acid excretion by the kidneys is impaired for two reasons. First, aldosterone stimulates H^+ secretion by the intercalated cells of the collecting ducts. In the absence of aldosterone, H^+ secretion at this site will be diminished, and less H^+ will be excreted.

Second, hyperkalemia inhibits ammoniagenesis by cells of the proximal tubule. Because ammonia is an important buffer, a reduction in its availability will contribute to the impairment of net acid excretion. (See pp. 801-804 in *Physiology* 3rd ed.)

Case 6

1. The acid-base disorder of this man is a metabolic acidosis. In the absence of insulin the metabolism of fats and carbohydrates is altered such that nonvolatile acids (ketoacids) are produced. The nonvolatile acids are rapidly buffered by cellular and extracellular buffers. Buffering in the extracellular fluid decreases the plasma $[HCO_3^-]$. The deep rapid breathing reflects the respiratory compensation (P_{CO_2} is lowered). (See pp. 798-799 and 804-806 in *Physiology* 3rd ed.)

2. Hyperkalemia in this patient is a result of a shift of K^+ out of cells (e.g., skeletal muscle) into the extracellular fluid. This shift occurs because of the lack of insulin and the hypertonicity of the ECF secondary to the elevated [glucose]. The acidosis is probably not a major contributing factor to the development of hyperkalemia in this situation. When acidosis is induced by mineral acids (e.g., HCl), movement of H^+ into cells during the process of intracellular buffering results in a shift of K^+ out of the cell and into the ECF. However, with organic acidosis, as occurs in this situation, the cellular buffering of the organic acids does not shift a significant amount of K^+ out of the cell. (See pp. 784-786 in *Physiology* 3rd ed.)

3. Insulin causes K^+ to move into cells. The mechanism responsible for this effect of insulin appears to be related to stimulation of the Na^+, K^+-ATPase. With increased activity of the Na^+, K^+-ATPase, K^+ uptake into the cell is enhanced. In addition, insulin's effect on glucose metabolism will lower the serum [glucose]. As a consequence, the osmolality of the ECF will decrease and cause additional K^+ to move into cells. (See pp. 785-786 in *Physiology* 3rd ed.)

4. The administration of HCO_3^- would increase the blood pH and shift some K^+ into cells. The HCO_3^- containing intravenous fluid would also increase the volume of the ECF and dilute the K^+ in this compartment. Studies in experimental animals have shown that the dilution of K^+ by expansion of the ECF is the primary mechanism by which the infusion of an HCO_3^--containing solution decreases the serum $[K^+]$. (See p. 785 in *Physiology* 3rd ed.)

5. The polyuria is a result of an osmotic diuresis induced by glucose. When the filtered load of glucose is below the T_m for glucose reabsorption in the proximal tubule, all of the filtered glucose is reabsorbed. However, in this man the filtered load of glucose will exceed the glucose T_m. Consequently, the nonreabsorbed glucose (filtered load - T_m) will remain in the lumen of the proximal tubule where it will act as an osmotically active particle. As NaCl and water are reabsorbed by the proximal tubule, the concentration of the nonreabsorbed glucose will increase. With this increase in concentration, an osmotic gradient opposite to that generated by the NaCl reabsorptive process is developed. Because proximal tubule reabsorption is isosmotic, the presence of this glucose osmotic gradient will inhibit a portion of proximal tubule NaCl and water reabsorption. Because of the glucose-induced osmotic diuresis, delivery of NaCl and water will be increased to the distal tubule and collecting duct, which will stimulate K^+ secretion at these sites. As a result, K^+ excretion from the body will be increased. Increased K^+ excretion together with the shift of K^+ from the ICF to the ECF secondary to the insulin deficiency and hyperosmolality will lead to progressive depletion of whole body K^+. Accordingly, an increase in serum $[K^+]$ is not always indicative of positive K^+ balance. This man is in negative K^+ balance, and is at risk of the development of hypokalemia when insulin is administered and the metabolic abnormalities are corrected. (See pp. 741-745, 749-751, and 788-791 in *Physiology* 3rd ed.)

6. The glucose-induced osmotic diuresis causes a loss of water from the body in excess of solute. This may lead to the development of hypernatremia. However, the hyperglycemia causes a shift of water from the ICF to the ECF, which dilutes the ECF Na^+. As therapy is initiated and the hyperglycemia is corrected, water will move back into the ICF and thereby lead to the development of hypernatremia. (See pp. 756-758 in *Physiology* 3rd ed.)

CHAPTER 44

1. The apparent loss of action of a peptide hormone in this patient could result from:
   a. An inability to secrete an adequate amount of the peptide hormone in question. (See pp. 815-818 in *Physiology* 3rd ed.)

   b. A loss of recognition of the hormone signal by the target cells of the hormone. (See pp. 80 and 819 in *Physiology* 3rd ed.)

   c. A loss of the signal transduction mechanism that ultimately stimulates the intracellular action of the hormone. (See pp. 81-85 and 818-825 in *Physiology* 3rd ed.)

2. Inability to secrete a peptide hormone could be the consequence of a number of possible defects. The endocrine cell may have lost its ability to recognize the stimulus for the secretion of the stored peptide hormone. An example would be a deficiency in the enzyme glucokinase, which is required for the recognition of elevated plasma glucose levels as a stimulus for the secretion of insulin by pancreatic islet beta cells. Another defect could lie in the gene for synthesis of the hormone that could have a nonsense or missense mutation in the hormone sequence. A nonsense mutation would lead to complete loss of production of any authentic hormone molecules. A missense mutation would lead to production of a hormone sequence, the structure of which might be altered enough to decrease the biologic activity of the hormone. The primary transcript of the hormone gene, that is, the preprohormone, could be mutated in an area that is critical for processing the preprohormone to the hormone. If so, the hormone molecule might not be cleaved normally from its precursor nor released to act on its target cells. An example would be a mutated proinsulin molecule or preproparathyroid hormone molecule. (See pp. 815-817, 854, 856, and 857 in *Physiology* 3rd ed.)

   Peptide hormones act through plasma membrane receptors with various domains. A gene mutation could give rise to various types of abnormalities in the hormone receptor. If the extracellular portion of the receptor were abnormal, binding of the hormone would be deficient because of a low affinity to the receptor. If a transmembrane loop of the receptor were abnormal, it might not interact properly with an adjacent signal transducer molecule. If the intracellular tail of the receptor were abnormal, an ATP binding site or tyrosine kinase active site could be abnormal and fail to carry out the hormone's action. Because receptor molecules also arise from a prorreceptor, a processing error could occur that would yield a total receptor deficiency. (See pp. 80, 821, 861, and 862 in *Physiology* 3rd ed.)

   Another genetic error that could lead to defective hormone action would be in transcription of a mutant G-protein. Such a mutant G-protein could fail to activate second messenger pathways such as adenylyl cyclase-cAMP. (See pp. 81-82 and 821-822 in *Physiology* 3rd ed.)

   Finally, a genetic error could lead to reduced synthesis of an enzyme that was a key element in the ultimate intracellular action of a hormone. (See p. 869 in *Physiology* 3rd ed.)

3. If deficient synthesis of the hormone were the problem, basal plasma levels of the hormone measured by radioimmunoassay would be low. Furthermore, the plasma hormone level would not rise in response to normal physiologic stimulation. If authentic hormone were administered to the patient, a normal response should occur. (See pp. 828-830 in *Physiology* 3rd ed.)

   On the other hand, if an abnormal hormone molecule were being synthesized and released, plasma levels might well be elevated, as measured by radioimmunoassay. This is because an assay antibody might still recognize portions of the abnormal molecule, and negative feedback from lack of hormone action would stimulate hormone secretions. However, if plasma hormone levels were measured by a biologic assay, the plasma levels would be low. If authentic hormone were administered in this situation, the patient still should respond normally. If processing of a preprohormone were defective, plasma levels of the preprohormone would be elevated, whereas plasma levels of the hormone itself would be low. (See pp. 817-818 and 828-830 in *Physiology* 3rd ed.)

In all situations where the defect in hormone action lies at the receptor step, plasma levels of the hormone should be very high because of negative feedback. If a preparation of the patient's receptor from available cells, such as white blood cells, were reacted with radioactively labeled hormone in vitro, the response curve would be shifted to the right; such a shift indicates a receptor with decreased affinity. If authentic hormone were administered to the patient, the physiologic response would be less than normal. (See pp. 817-818, 820-821, and 826-827 in *Physiology* 3rd ed.)

In situations where the block in hormone action was downstream from the receptor step, plasma hormone levels again should be high. However, preparations of the patient's receptor would bind radioactively labeled hormone molecules normally in vitro. On the other hand, preparations of target cells from the patient would fail to exhibit either increases in second messenger levels (e.g., cAMP hormone) or normal increases in metabolic products of hormone action (e.g., glycogen), when incubated with the hormone.

4. After studies of the type just mentioned, the likely site of biologic hormone deficiency should be pinpointed. The appropriate gene (hormone, receptor, G-protein, or target enzyme) should be cloned from the patient and its structure compared with that of the normal gene. The same genes from the two parents and all siblings should be cloned. Because the inheritance pattern appears to be autosomal recessive, each parent would be expected to have one normal allele for the gene in question and one abnormal allele like that of the patient. The patient should have two abnormal alleles. Any sibling with one mutant allele would be identified as a carrier for this defect in hormone action and suitably counseled when at a reproductive age.

5. In an autosomal recessive disease, one-fourth of the siblings will have two normal alleles (one from each parent) for the gene in question and hence will be disease free. Siblings with only one mutant allele are like the parents. The presence of one normal allele is enough to direct sufficient synthesis of the normal hormone, receptor, or G-protein to allow for a normal biologic state with only 50% of the normal concentration. This would imply that the mutant gene product does not inhibit the action of the normal gene product (as is the case in some instances).

CHAPTER 45

1. A typical, healthy adult man in the resting basal state expends approximately 20 kcal/kg, which equals 1400 kcal/day in this person. Ordinary spontaneous movements would account for another 300 to 400 kcal/day. His 1 hour of exercise would require approximately 250 kcal. Thus his total daily energy expenditure might be approximately 2000 kcal initially. As fasting continued, his basal metabolic rate would diminish about 15% to approximately 1200 kcal/day and lethargy might also reduce both spontaneous and voluntary physical movement. Thus, for the 4 weeks, his overall energy expenditure could average 1800 kcal/day. (See pp. 834 and 846 in *Physiology* 3rd ed.)

2. His total caloric needs for 28 days would be 56,000 endogenous kcal (1800 per day x 28 days). Ninety percent of this would be supplied by fat at 9 kcal/g. Thus, 0.9 x 56,000 ÷ 9 equals 5600 g or 5.6 kg of fat. Adipose tissue is composed of 15% water. Hence, 5.6 ÷ 0.85 or 6.6 kg of adipose tissue would be lost. Ten percent of the caloric needs would be supplied by protein at 4 kcal/g. Thus, 0.1 x 56,000 ÷ 4 equals 1400 g or 1.4 kg of protein that would be lost. The source of this protein is lean body mass, which is composed of 72% water. Thus, 1.4 ÷ 0.28, or 5 kg, of lean body mass would be lost. Carbohydrate stores of energy are very low and contribute no more than 0.3 to 0.4 kg, all in the first 2 days. Thus the estimated total weight loss would be 6.6 plus 5, plus 0.4, or 12 kg. His respiratory quotient would be slightly greater than 0.7 because of the predominance of fat as a substrate for oxidation. (See pp. 834, 836, 846, and 847 in *Physiology* 3rd ed.)

3. Plasma glucose would decrease to a lower, but stable level after glycogen stores were depleted. Plasma free fatty acids and glycerol would increase because of accelerated lipolysis, and keto acids (beta-hydroxybutyrate and acetoacetate) would increase as a result of increased free fatty acid delivery to the liver. Plasma branch chain amino acids would increase because of increased proteolysis in muscle. Urinary nitrogen would increase, indicating degradation of endogenous protein. Excretion of sodium in the urine would promptly cease in the absence of sodium intake after a small fall in extracellular fluid volume. Excretion of the predominantly intracellular electrolytes (potassium and phosphate) would continue, indicating the loss of protoplasm. (See pp. 775, 839-841, and 847 in *Physiology* 3rd ed.)

4. Initially, the brain would be almost entirely dependent on glucose generated by gluconeogenesis, mostly from amino acid substrates liberated by muscle proteolysis. Gradually, however, keto acids generated by oxidation of free fatty acids would become brain substrates and would eventually supply two thirds of the brain's energy needs. This would help to conserve lean body mass during fasting. (See pp. 839, 840, and 846 in *Physiology* 3rd ed.)

5. Plasma insulin would decrease and plasma glucagon would increase. The lower ratio of insulin to glucagon facilitates mobilization of liver glycogen, adipose tissue triglycerides, and muscle protein. (See pp. 847 and 870-871 in *Physiology* 3rd ed.)

6. Serum thyroid-stimulating hormone (TSH) and its response to thyrotropin-releasing hormone (TRH) would decrease. In addition, serum triiodothyronine (T_3) would decrease because of reduced 5' monodeiodination of thyroxine (T_4). The net result is a lower level of the active T_3 molecule, which contributes to the decrease in resting energy expenditure. Cortisol secretion would increase modestly, facilitating muscle proteolysis and gluconeogenesis. Growth hormone levels increase, facilitating lipolysis. However, conversion of growth hormone to somatomedin would be greatly diminished. The loss of somatomedin's stimulation of protein synthesis shunts amino acids away from anabolic storage toward conversion to needed glucose. Maintenance of cortisol and elevated growth hormone levels

diminishes the sensitivity of muscle to insulin and further preserves the glucose supply to the brain. (See pp. 904, 917-920, 940-947, and 959-962 in *Physiology* 3rd ed.)

7.   Ingestion of any source of carbohydrate would raise plasma glucose and thereby rapidly stimulate insulin release and inhibit glucagon and growth hormone release. Glucose oxidation would increase and thus raise the respiratory quotient. Storage of glucose as glycogen in liver and muscle would be stimulated by insulin. At the same time, uptake of potassium and phosphate by these tissues would be stimulated, causing a decrease in their plasma levels. A sharp decrease in plasma free fatty acids, keto acids, and branch chain amino acids would be expected as the high insulin levels reduced lipolysis, ketogenesis, and proteolysis. (See pp. 785, 836, 865, 915, 916, and 968 in *Physiology* 3rd ed.)

CHAPTER 46

1. The primary cause is *insulin deficiency* resulting from destruction of the beta cells of the pancreatic islets. Secondarily, loss of insulin leads to disinhibition of glucagon secretion by the alpha cells of the islets, and thereby causes *glucagon excess*. The clinical consequences of insulin deficiency and glucagon excess create a state of "stress," which additionally stimulates *cortisol* secretion, *growth hormone* secretion, and *epinephrine* and *norepinephrine* release. This complete hormonal setting of insulin deficiency arrayed against increases of glucagon, cortisol, growth hormone, and catecholamines generates hyperglycemia. (See pp. 851-854 and 868 in *Physiology* 3rd ed.)

2. Hepatic glucose production and release are elevated, initially because of exaggerated glycogen breakdown (low insulin, high glucagon, high epinephrine) and subsequently because of increased rates of gluconeogenesis (high glucagon, cortisol, catecholamines, low insulin). The efficiency of glucose uptake by both muscle and adipose tissue is diminished because of impaired glucose transport and intracellular blocks in glucose metabolism (low insulin, high cortisol, high epinephrine). The high plasma glucose level is required to maintain normal rates of intracellular glucose utilization. Finally, as dehydration occurs, plasma glucose rises still further because of a reduction in glomerular filtration rate. (See pp. 859, 868, 959, and 974 in *Physiology* 3rd ed.)

3. The bidirectional flow between glucose and phosphoenolpyruvate is determined by the bidirectional flow between fructose-6-phosphate and fructose-1,6-biphosphate. These two phosphates in turn are modulated by the level of fructose-2,6-biphosphate. A low ratio of insulin to glucagon decreases the level of fructose-2,6-biphosphate, which increases flow toward fructose-6-phosphate and gluconeogenesis by activating fructose-1,6-biphosphatase and inhibiting 6-phosphofructokinase. Flow from phosphoenolpyruvate to pyruvate (glycolysis) is determined by the activity of pyruvate kinase, which is diminished by insulin deficiency. Flow from pyruvate to phosphoenolpyruvate (gluconeogenesis) is determined by pyruvate carboxylase and phosphoenolpyruvate carboxykinase, which are increased by high cortisol and glucagon levels and low insulin levels. In brief, the hormonally induced alterations in this patient at key control points favor gluconeogenesis over glycolysis and glucose production over its utilization. (See pp. 864, 869, and 870 in *Physiology* 3rd ed.)

4. Deficiency of insulin plus excess of catecholamines, glucagon, growth hormone, and cortisol generates unrestrained lipolysis of adipose tissue triglycerides. The increased flow of free fatty acids to the liver greatly exceeds that organ's oxidative capacity. Large quantities of four carbon ketoacids are formed (beta hydroxybutyrate and acetoacetate) and released by the liver. These acids have pK values well below 6.1 and require buffering by sodium bicarbonate This reaction produces the sodium salts of the keto acids and carbonic acid. The latter dissociates to carbon dioxide and water. (See p. 864 in *Physiology* 3rd ed.)

5. Excess production of CO_2 stimulates central chemoreceptors and peripheral chemoreceptors by increasing extracellular hydrogen ion concentrations. This increases the rate of ventilation. However, the resultant fall in the Pa_{CO_2} produced by this patient's maximum respiratory effort failed to compensate for the marked reduction in plasma bicarbonate. According to the Henderson-Hasselbach equation, an increase in blood hydrogen ion concentration occurs, that is, a fall in pH. (See pp. 602, 603, and 798 in *Physiology* 3rd ed.)

6. For 6 weeks, high plasma glucose levels created a filtered load of glucose that exceeded the tubular maximum for renal tubular glucose reabsorption. The glucose that escaped reabsorption caused an osmotic diuresis. This, along with the lessened oral intake of water and the gastrointestinal losses from

vomiting, resulted in severe dehydration and hypovolemia that lowered the blood pressure. In turn, decreased baroreceptor firing caused a reflex tachycardia. (See p. 538 in *Physiology* 3rd ed.)

7. Plasma free fatty acids will be high because of increased lipolysis. Plasma triglycerides will be high because of increased production of very low density lipoprotein from the increased free fatty acid load to the liver. This elevation of triglycerides will be aggravated by decreased clearance of very low density lipoprotein from plasma because of loss of adipose tissue lipoprotein lipase activity when insulin is deficient. (See pp. 864-865 in *Physiology* 3rd ed.)

8. Plasma branch chain amino acids will be high because of increased muscle proteolysis in the absence of insulin and because of elevated cortisol levels. The high amino acid flow to the liver sustains accelerated rates of gluconeogenesis. (See pp. 839-840, 842, and 961 in *Physiology* 3rd ed.)

9. Plasma aldosterone will be high, stimulated by the renin-angiotensin system, which is activated by the patient's hypovolemia. Plasma antidiuretic hormones (ADH) will be high, mostly stimulated by a high plasma osmolality from glucose and secondarily by hypovolemia. (See pp. 925-926, 966, and 967 in *Physiology* 3rd ed.)

10. There are three components to the patient's weight loss: (a) extracellular fluid losses from osmotic diuresis and vomiting; (b) loss of adipose mass because insulin deficiency leads to increased lipolysis and decreased reesterification of free fatty acids by glycerol phosphate; and (c) loss of lean body mass because insulin deficiency accelerates proteolysis and diminishes protein synthesis. In addition, somatomedin levels fall, further decreasing protein synthesis. (See p. 864 in *Physiology* 3rd ed.)

11. High plasma osmolality plus hypovolemia stimulates thirst. Appetite increases in response to wasting large quantities of calories as glucose in the urine. (See p. 762 in *Physiology* 3rd ed.)

12. Urea nitrogen excretion will be elevated, reflecting high rates of amino acid use for gluconeogenesis instead of for protein synthesis. Ammonia excretion will be elevated as a means of buffering excess hydrogen ion generated by the presence of strong ketoacids in the tubular urine. Potassium phosphate and magnesium excretion will be increased because these intracellular electrolytes are released when glycogen and protein stores diminish. (See pp. 802-804 in *Physiology* 3rd ed.)

13. Restoration of insulin will inhibit lipolysis and reduce production of the strong ketoacids. This will result in an increase in plasma bicarbonate and pH. Plasma potassium will fall for several reasons: (a) insulin directly stimulates potassium uptake by cells; (b) as insulin diminishes ketoacid levels and extracellular fluid acidosis, potassium will move from extracellular fluid to intracellular fluid in exchange for hydrogen ion released from intracellular buffers; and (c) as insulin decreases plasma glucose, water will move from extracellular space to the intracellular space, and potassium will be carried along by solvent drag. Plasma phosphate will fall because insulin stimulates cellular uptake of phosphate as glucose transport is increased and phosphorylated glucose intermediates are formed. (See p. 865 in *Physiology* 3rd ed.)

CHAPTER 47

1. Total plasma calcium consists of a protein-bound (approximately 50%) and an ionized portion (approximately 50%). An increase above normal in plasma albumin of 1 g/dl, as in this patient, could account for a 0.8 mg/dl increase in the total plasma calcium level without increasing the biologically active ionized calcium level. To be certain that the ionized calcium level is increased, it must be measured directly. (See p. 876 in *Physiology* 3rd ed.)

2. The most likely hormonal causes are vitamin D, 1,25-$(OH)_2$-vitamin D, PTH, and PTHrp. T_4 and certain lymphokines and cytokines are less common causes. (See pp. 884 and 888 in *Physiology* 3rd ed.)

3. If excess vitamin D were ingested, this would be converted to 24-OH-vitamin D and hence to 1,25-$(OH)_2$-vitamin D. The latter active metabolite of vitamin D primarily increases calcium absorption from the gut. A second effect is to increase bone resorption. PTH might be secreted in excess by an enlarged neoplastic parathyroid gland. PTH increases reabsorption of calcium from the distal renal tubules; PTH directly stimulates resorption of bone; PTH stimulates renal production of 1,25-$(OH)_2$-vitamin D from 25-OH-vitamin D by activating the 1-hydroxylase enzyme and it leads to an increased absorption of calcium from the gut. PTHrp, a larger molecule with an N-terminal amino acid sequence identical to PTH, is secreted by a variety of tumors. This molecule mimics all the above actions of PTH by interacting with the PTH receptor. T_4 and cytokines, such as interleukin-1 and tumor necrosis factor, stimulate bone resorption. (See pp. 884, 885, and 887-891 in *Physiology* 3rd ed.)

4. The low plasma phosphate suggests PTH or PTHrp as the causes of the hypercalcemia. Both molecules increase urinary phosphate excretion by inhibiting reabsorption of phosphate in the proximal renal tubules. This keeps plasma phosphate low. In contrast, 1,25-$(OH)_2$-vitamin D, lymphokines and cytokines, and T_4 all increase entry of phosphate into the plasma by stimulating bone resorption; thus plasma phosphate tends to rise. (See p. 889 in *Physiology* 3rd ed.)

5. An excess of 1,25-$(OH)_2$-vitamin D would decrease the plasma PTH level by negative feedback from the hypercalcemia and also by direct repression of transcription of the PTH gene. An excess of PTH would increase plasma 1,25-$(OH)_2$-vitamin D by stimulating its production (see preceding answer). An excess of PTHrp would decrease plasma PTH by negative feedback from the hypercalcemia; 1,25-$(OH)_2$-vitamin D would remain normal or increase depending on the affinity of the renal tubular PTH receptor for PTHrp. T_4, cytokines, and lymphokines would decrease plasma PTH by negative feedback from the hypercalcemia. Some cytokines might increase 1,25-$(OH)_2$-vitamin D levels by stimulating its synthesis within mononuclear cells. (See p. 887 in *Physiology* 3rd ed.)

6. Excess PTH secretion elevates plasma calcium. As long as the glomerular filtration rate remains normal, this elevation increases the filtered load of calcium enough to saturate tubular reabsorption mechanisms and to increase calcium concentration in the urine. If the solubility product of calcium oxalate is exceeded, crystals form and aggregate into renal stones. (See p. 895 in *Physiology* 3rd ed.)

7. Excess PTH stimulates osteoclasts to enlarge, change their shape, and release enzymes that digest bone completely. Pain is associated with weakened bone structure resulting from the accelerated bone reabsorption. The products of collagen breakdown yield increased amounts of hydroxyproline in the urine. Bone formation by osteoblasts is normally coupled to bone resorption; therefore bone formation also increases, and this is indicated by an elevated plasma alkaline phosphatase. (See pp. 879-880 and 888 in *Physiology* 3rd ed.)

8. Calcium and sodium share renal tubular reabsorption mechanisms. A high filtered load of calcium decreases sodium reabsorption and causes an osmotic diuresis and polyuria. In addition, high calcium levels inhibit renal responses to ADH. In hyperparathyroidism, urinary cyclic AMP excretion is increased because cyclic AMP is the second messenger for PTH. (See pp. 887 and 889 in *Physiology* 3rd ed.)

9. A sharp fall in plasma calcium could result from previous suppression of the uninvolved normal parathyroid glands by hypercalcemia or from their damage during surgery. In this case, plasma PTH would be low and plasma phosphate would be high because of the loss of the inhibitory effect of PTH on renal phosphate reabsorption. Alternatively, the fall in plasma calcium could result from a sudden cessation of excessive rates of bone resorption caused by the high PTH levels. Excessive bone formation could, however, continue until the coupling mechanism restored it to normal. During this period of rebuilding bone, calcium uptake by bone would exceed calcium release from bone, so that plasma calcium would tend to be low. Plasma PTH would be high because of negative feedback. Plasma phosphate would be low because phosphate is also required for bone formation; therefore its uptake by bone would exceed its release from bone. In addition, the secondarily elevated PTH level would stimulate urinary phosphate excretion. (See pp. 887-890 in *Physiology* 3rd ed.)

10. Hyperventilation would lead to hypocapnia and respiratory alkalosis. The increase in pH would increase calcium binding to plasma protein, and thereby lower the biologically active ionized fraction of calcium. This can produce neuromuscular irritability with muscle spasms (tetany) and abnormal sensations (paresthesias). (See pp. 806 and 876 in *Physiology* 3rd ed.)

CHAPTER 48

Case 1

1. The features of this patient and the history of the changes in his appearance and shoe size strongly suggest an excess of growth hormone (GH). This is usually caused by a tumor of pituitary somatotrophs, and this disease is called acromegaly. (See pp. 914 and 919 in *Physiology* 3rd ed.)

2. GH stimulates the synthesis of a peptide mediator called somatomedin or insulin-like growth factor-1 (IGF-1). This is produced in the liver, but also in many other tissues that contain GH target cells. Plasma somatomedin levels will be high in patients with GH-secreting tumors. (See pp. 918-919 in *Physiology* 3rd ed.)

3. GH via somatomedin (and its plasma membrane receptor) stimulates proliferation of chondrocytes (cartilage cells), osteoblasts and connective tissue cells. This causes excess linear growth in children and giantism results. In adults whose bone growth centers are already closed, appositional bone growth is stimulated. This causes widening of digits, thickened vertebrae, ribs, skull bones, and mandible, with resultant alteration in facial features and position of the teeth. Proliferation of muscle cells increases lean body mass, as exemplified by enlargement of the muscular tongue. The visceral parenchymal cell growth is stimulated, which causes enlargement of organs such as the liver and kidneys. (See pp. 878, 917, and 918 in *Physiology* 3rd ed.)

4. Stimulation of the growth of connective tissue and synovium and cartilage causes osteoarthritis. Also, nerves can be compressed by the growing bone at points where the nerves pass through grooves in the bone. (See p. 917 in *Physiology* 3rd ed.)

5. Glucose normally suppresses GH release. When GH is created autonomously by a somatotrophic tumor, there is usually no response to glucose administration. (See pp. 915-917 in *Physiology* 3rd ed.)

6. GH is an insulin antagonistic hormone that inhibits insulin-stimulated glucose uptake by muscle cells as well as the insulin effects on the liver. Thus the fasting plasma glucose level rises. In response to the high glucose levels, plasma insulin levels will also be elevated. In addition, GH directly stimulates growth of pancreatic islet beta cells. (See p. 918 in *Physiology* 3rd ed.)

7. There are three possible causes of the patient's impotence, which reflect a low plasma testosterone level. First, the pituitary tumor may have destroyed gonadotropin-producing cells by exerting pressure on them. The resultant loss of luteinizing hormone (LH) and follicle-stimulating hormone (FSH) decreases the secretion of testosterone by the Leydig cells of the testes. Second, the tumor may have compressed the hypophyseal stalk and cut off transport of gonadotropin-releasing hormone (GnRH) down the pituitary portal veins from the median eminence to the anterior pituitary gonadotrophs; this process would decrease LH and FSH secretions. Third, such tumors may secrete prolactin, a hormone structurally related to GH. High prolactin levels inhibit GnRH release from the hypothalamus and thus would decrease LH and FSH secretion. (See pp. 899, 913, 914, 920, 985, 986, and 1000 in *Physiology* 3rd ed.)

8. Similarly, ACTH and/or TSH secretion might be impaired by the same two mechanisms described above for LH and FSH. This would in turn cause cortisol and thyroxine deficiencies.

9. The optic nerves cross just above the pituitary gland on their route to the occipital cortex. Pressure from a tumor on this crossing point causes a characteristic defect in the visual fields. (See pp. 156-158 in *Physiology* 3rd ed.)

10. Growth hormone secretion is normally under dual regulation from the hypothalamus. It is stimulated by GnRH and inhibited by somatostatin. The latter, in a long-acting analog form, can reduce the elevated GH levels in patients with acromegaly because their tumors contain plasma membrane receptors for the hypothalamic inhibitory peptide. (See pp. 915-917 in *Physiology* 3rd ed.)

11. The swelling of soft tissues would resolve promptly. However, the bone changes caused by excess GH would resolve very slowly (and perhaps not at all) because of the relatively slow rate of normal bone turnover. (See pp. 878-881 in *Physiology* 3rd ed.)

12. Inadvertent removal of the anterior pituitary gland would cause permanent deficiencies of TSH, ACTH, FSH, LH, MSH, and prolactin. Replacement therapy with thyroxine and cortisol would be necessary. Aldosterone would not be needed because its secretion would be maintained by the renin-angiotensin system. Lack of MSH action might cause pale skin and the inability to get a tan upon exposure to ultraviolet light. There are no known consequences of prolactin deficiency in males. Removal of the posterior pituitary gland would not ordinarily cause ADH deficiency as long as the suprahypophyseal portion of the axons from the hypothalamic neurons that synthesize ADH remained intact. (See pp. 899, 909, 910, 924, 966, and 967 in *Physiology* 3rd ed.)

13. If the patient still wished to father a child, and his gonadotrophic cells were not significantly damaged, then treatment with daily pulsatile administration of GnRH would be effective. If his gonadotrophic cells were destroyed, he would require regular administration of LH and FSH. If the patient only wished to restore sexual potency, he would require only testosterone replacement therapy. (See p. 1000 in *Physiology* 3rd ed.)

Case 2

1. A urine osmolality consistently lower than plasma osmolality indicates a high rate of clearance of free, osmotically unencumbered water. It could be a normal compensation for an excessive voluntary intake of water, or it could indicate an inability of the patient's kidneys to reabsorb water and concentrate the urine. The latter defect could be caused by an intrinsic renal abnormality or a lack of the necessary signal(s) to the kidneys to conserve water. (See p. 769 in *Physiology* 3rd ed.)

2. Sodium and its associated anions constitute the predominant solute in plasma water. An elevated concentration of sodium generally indicates a deficit of total body water, because extracellular fluid and intracellular fluid are in osmotic equilibrium. Because sodium cannot enter cells to any great extent, the absolute plasma sodium level is also an excellent quantitative indicator of the magnitude of the body water deficit. The percentage increase in serum sodium above normal is equivalent to the percentage decrease in total body water, providing there has been no significant loss of sodium itself from the body. (See pp. 755-758 in *Physiology* 3rd ed.)

3. Tubular urine is isosmotic until it reaches the loop of Henle. The operation of the countercurrent multiplication system (passive rapid reabsorption of water in the thin descending limb and active reabsorption of sodium in the thick ascending limb) produces a hyperosmotic medullary interstitial fluid. When the resultant hypoosmotic distal tubular fluid reaches the collecting ducts, water is reabsorbed because of the large osmotic gradient between the tubular lumen and the interstitial fluid.

Reabsorption occurs through cell membranes whose permeability to water is physiologically modulated to increase flow from tubular lumen into the cell when water conservation is necessary. (See pp. 764-770 in *Physiology* 3rd ed.)

4. A single hormone, ADH, stimulates the process of water conservation, and the product is a final urine that is hyperosmotic to plasma. ADH acts on the thick ascending limb of the loop of Henle to stimulate sodium reabsorption. Most important, however, ADH increases the permeability of the collecting duct cell to water. ADH acts through cyclic AMP as a second messenger. Membrane proteins are phosphorylated, and subsequently water-conveying cytoplasmic organelles move to and fuse with the luminal side of the plasma membrane. Once water has entered the cell, it is drawn into the medullary interstitium by the high osmolarity generated by the countercurrent multiplication system. The urine/plasma osmolality ratio can reach a maximum of 4:1. (See pp. 760-762, 766, 767, 927, and 928 in *Physiology* 3rd ed.)

5. ADH is synthesized from a large precursor molecule in hypothalamic neurons in the supraoptic and paraventricular nuclei. ADH travels down the axons and is stored in granules in the posterior pituitary gland. From there, ADH is released by exocytosis after a nerve impulse causes calcium influx into the granules. (See pp. 899 and 923-924 in *Physiology* 3rd ed.)

6. ADH is released in response to an increase in plasma osmolality caused by any substance, such as sodium, which cannot readily enter cells. Thus, plasma hyperosmolality, resulting from the loss of free water, stimulates osmoreceptor cells in the hypothalamus; these in turn stimulate ADH secretory neurons. A decrease in blood volume and pressure also stimulates ADH release via baroreceptor and other stretch reflexes. Other nonspecific stimuli of ADH release include pain, nausea, and psychic stress. (See pp. 924-926 in *Physiology* 3rd ed.)

7. a. The skull fracture could have disrupted the patient's thirst mechanism and caused primary polydipsia. However, in that case, the patient's plasma sodium and osmolality would have been decreased rather than increased. Furthermore, when she was subjected to water deprivation, her urine volume would have decreased normally to 30 to 50 ml/hr.

   b. Unsuspected renal trauma could have caused a tubular insensitivity to the action of ADH; this is called nephrogenic diabetes insipidus. However, this is unlikely, given that there were no red blood cells in the urine and the patient's serum creatinine and blood urea nitrogen levels were normal.

   c. The skull fracture could have caused structural or functional damage to the mechanism for releasing ADH. This is called central diabetes insipidus. ADH deficiency is the most likely explanation for the patient's polyuria and thirst. (See p. 929 in *Physiology* 3rd ed.)

8. The patient's plasma level of ADH was almost certainly low. This could reflect destruction or damage to the ADH secretory neurons or damage to osmoreceptor cells, with an upward resetting of the osmostat for ADH release. The plasma ADH level would also have been low after damage to the thirst mechanism, because the excess water intake would have suppressed ADH secretion by negative feedback from a decrease in plasma osmolality and an increase in circulating volume. In the case of renal tubular damage, the plasma ADH level would be elevated by the constant state of water deficiency. (See p. 925 in *Physiology* 3rd ed.)

9. Administration of ADH to the patient would sharply reduce the rate of urine flow by reducing free water clearance. As plasma osmolality declines to normal, thirst would diminish. This response would

help to confirm the diagnosis of central diabetes insipidus. If renal tubular insensitivity to ADH were the fundamental problem, the administration of ADH would have little or no effect on the rate of urine flow. (See pp. 762 and 927 in *Physiology* 3rd ed.)

10. The patient had ADH deficiency, which is referred to as central diabetes insipidus. (See p. 929 in *Physiology* 3rd ed.)

11. The patient should be taught to administer ADH when she notes the return of a high urine flow rate. If she waits for a return of thirst as a signal, she will always be slightly water deprived because thirst would indicate a significant rise in plasma osmolality. (See pp. 762 and 929 in *Physiology* 3rd ed.)

12. A higher dietary intake of sodium or a higher intake of protein (which generates urea) would increase the osmolar load. This would create a higher rate of delivery of fluid to the distal nephron. In turn, this would decrease the osmolar gradient between the distal tubular urine and the medullary interstitium. Thus, less water would be reabsorbed even in the presence of ADH, and urine volume would increase. (See p. 765 in *Physiology* 3rd ed.)

13. When a patient with central diabetes insipidus is stuporous, thirst is inoperative. This condition places both water intake and water output in the hands of the physician. If too much fluid is given intravenously along with effective doses of ADH, water retention may become excessive and serious hypoosmolality may result. This state of water intoxication can lead to further central nervous system dysfunction and even convulsions. (See p. 929 in *Physiology* 3rd ed.)

CHAPTER 49

1. Loss of weight despite normal food intake indicates negative caloric balance caused by energy expenditure exceeding energy intake. An excess level of thyroid hormone has increased the patient's basal or resting metabolic rate, that is, the rate of oxygen utilization above normal. In addition, thyroid hormone excess has caused a negative nitrogen balance, with the rate of protein degradation exceeding the rate of protein synthesis, so that lean body mass and bone mass have declined along with adipose tissue. The high basal metabolic rate induced by thyroid hormone is accompanied by increased heat production, which causes intolerance to high environmental temperatures and stimulates mechanisms of heat loss, such as sweating and hyperventilation. Nervousness, tremor, rapid reflexes, and tachycardia reflect increased adrenergic nervous system activity. Muscle weakness is caused by a loss of muscle mass that results in enhanced proteolysis. Increased fatigability with exercise is caused by inefficient generation of ATP and reduced stores of creatine phosphate. The patient's cardiac output has been increased through thyroid hormone-induced increases in preload, cardiac contractility, and stroke volume. Systemic vascular resistance is decreased; this is attributable to local vasodilation caused by increased rates of tissue metabolism. (See pp. 254-256, 483, 518, 833, 834, 841, and 942-945 in *Physiology* 3rd ed.)

2. Enhanced expression of myosin heavy chain alpha genes and repression of myosin heavy chain beta genes increases the velocity of myocardial contraction. The increase in basal oxygen utilization is partly caused by enhanced expression of the Na^+, K^+-ATPase gene. Overactivity of the sympathetic nervous system is partly caused by enhanced expression of the beta adrenergic receptor gene. (See pp. 942 and 943 in *Physiology* 3rd ed.)

3. The serum T_3 level would be elevated. This is largely attributable to the high serum level of T_4, from which most T_3 is derived by peripheral conversion. To a lesser extent T_3 secretion is increased by the enlarged thyroid gland. T_3 is the active metabolite of T_4, and it binds with tenfold greater affinity to the nuclear thyroid hormone receptor. Therefore increased T_3 accounts for most of the patient's clinical signs. (See pp. 940 and 941 in *Physiology* 3rd ed.)

4. Excess secretion of thyroid hormone almost always results from disease intrinsic to the thyroid gland, and therefore such secretion is autonomous and independent of TSH stimulation of the gland. The resultant high serum T_4 and T_3 levels inhibit TSH secretion by blocking the effect of TRH on the pituitary thyrotrophs. The serum TSH level is therefore low. (See pp. 903-904 in *Physiology* 3rd ed.)

5. The serum TSH level would be elevated only in the rare case in which hypothyroidism was caused by excessive release of TRH or by secretion of TSH from a pituitary neoplasm.

6. Normal pregnancy is accompanied by high levels of estrogenic hormones. Estrogen increases the level of serum thyroid-binding globulin and therefore increases binding capacity. Consequently, total serum T_4 rises but free T_4 remains essentially normal, and the pregnant woman is basically euthyroid. The negative pregnancy test eliminates this consideration in the patient. In addition, the serum free T_4 was clearly elevated. (See p. 1017 in *Physiology* 3rd ed.)

7. An increased rate of synthesis of T_4 requires increased availability of iodide to the thyroid gland. If the total body pool of iodide stays normal, then a larger than normal percentage of that pool must be taken up by the thyroid gland each day to maintain a high level of thyroid hormone synthesis and release. (See p. 934 in *Physiology* 3rd ed.)

8. Thiouracil drugs inhibit the enzyme peroxidase, which catalyzes all steps in thyroid hormone synthesis from iodide and tyrosine. In addition to reducing T_4 synthesis and release, thiouracil drugs inhibit the enzyme 5' monodeiodinase and thereby decrease the peripheral production of T_3 from T_4. (See pp. 934, 935, 938, and 940 in *Physiology* 3rd ed.)

9. Although the thiouracil drug was initially beneficial, continued suppression of thyroid hormone synthesis produced a state of hypothyroidism. The basal metabolic rate decreased below normal, leading to inordinate weight gain. Cold intolerance resulted from subnormal thermogenesis. Bradycardia and lethargy resulted from diminished adrenergic nervous system activity. (See pp. 945 and 946 in *Physiology* 3rd ed.)

10. When the patient developed hypothyroidism, the operation of negative feedback caused an elevation in the serum level of TSH. Low serum T_4 and T_3 levels elicit overstimulation of the pituitary thyrotrophs by TRH. (See p. 903 in *Physiology* 3rd ed.)

11. The thyroid gland was initially enlarged because of hyperthyroidism (Graves' disease). The later reenlargement of the thyroid gland during thiouracil therapy reflected the trophic action of excess TSH acting through its thyroid plasma membrane receptor to stimulate DNA, RNA, and protein synthesis. (See p. 937 in *Physiology* 3rd ed.)

CHAPTER 50

Case 1

1. Given the elevated bicarbonate and reduced chloride and potassium levels, chronic metabolic alkalosis with respiratory compensation is the most likely acid-base disturbance in this patient. Arterial blood pH would be slightly increased; P_{CO_2} would also be increased. A much less likely diagnosis would be chronic respiratory acidosis with metabolic compensation. In that case, however, arterial blood pH would be decreased, and P_{CO_2} would be increased. (See pp. 805-806 in *Physiology* 3rd ed.)

2. a. Vomiting with loss of hydrogen ions (as hydrochloric acid) in gastric juice and return of the simultaneously generated bicarbonate to the extracellular fluid cause metabolic alkalosis. This is aggravated by enhanced renal tubular bicarbonate reabsorption secondary to contraction of the extracellular fluid. Renal potassium losses and hypokalemia are secondary to the metabolic alkalosis. (See pp. 661, 662, 790-791, 801, and 802 in *Physiology* 3rd ed.)

    b. Ingestion of a diuretic that inhibits proximal tubular sodium reabsorption increases sodium and water delivery to the distal tubular regions. This in turn enhances both potassium and hydrogen ion secretion, which results in hypokalemia and metabolic alkalosis. (See pp. 788-789 in *Physiology* 3rd ed.)

    c. Excess secretion of a mineralocorticoid hormone causes hypokalemia and metabolic alkalosis. (See p. 968 in *Physiology* 3rd ed.)

3. a. Loss of gastric juices is an unlikely cause in this patient because of the absence of vomiting. In addition, there were no signs of hypovolemia (low blood pressure, rapid heart rate) nor of a decrease in glomerular filtration rate (elevated plasma creatinine and blood urea nitrogen levels).

    b. Lack of signs of hypovolemia and a failure to correct the acid-base and electrolyte abnormalities on cessation of the diuretic are evidence that the drug did not cause the problem.

    c. An excess of a mineralocorticoid hormone is strongly suggested by the presence of hypertension and by the persistence of hypokalemia, despite administration of large amounts of potassium to the patient. (See pp. 968 and 969 in *Physiology* 3rd ed.)

    d. Lack of any history of pulmonary dysfunction and a decreased, rather than increased, respiratory rate is strong evidence against chronic respiratory acidosis. In addition, serum potassium would be expected to be high rather than low. (See p. 806 in *Physiology* 3rd ed.)

4. Measurement of potassium in the urine would be helpful. The presence of substantial amounts, greater than 40 mEq/day in the face of hypokalemia, would point to a renal tubular disturbance. Very small amounts of potassium in the urine would suggest that hypokalemia was caused by potassium loss in intestinal secretions. (See pp. 785-788 in *Physiology* 3rd ed.)

5. The adrenal mineralocorticoid hormone, aldosterone, and cortisol should be measured. Aldosterone should be measured when the patient is hypokalemic, in a sodium replete state, and in a recumbent position. These physiologic circumstances should normally inhibit aldosterone secretion. Therefore a high plasma level of aldosterone found in such circumstances suggests hyperaldosteronism. Plasma renin should then be measured to determine if the renin-angiotensin system is driving the pathologic

aldosterone excess. A high renin level suggests that unappreciated hypovolemia or constriction of a renal artery is the cause of the metabolic disturbance. A low renin level, particularly obtained when the patient is upright and in the sodium depleted condition (which should stimulate renin release), would argue for autonomous hypersecretion of aldosterone as the cause of the hypokalemia and metabolic alkalosis. (See pp. 772, 773, 966, and 967 in *Physiology* 3rd ed.)

6. An aldosterone excess stimulates sodium reabsorption and potassium secretion in the distal nephron. This causes expansion of extracellular fluid volume, hypertension, and hypokalemia. (See pp. 772, 774, and 788 in *Physiology* 3rd ed.)

7. Aldosterone binds to a nuclear receptor, and the complex induces expression of the Na^+, K^+-ATPase gene. This increases enzyme concentration in the basal membrane of the renal tubular cell. The action of Na^+, K^+-ATPase stimulates reentry of Na^+ into the plasma and secretion of K^+ into the tubular lumen. Hydrogen ion secretion is also directly stimulated. In addition, H^+ is transferred into the tubular lumen in response to the electronegative gradient created by Na^+ reabsorption. (See pp. 968-969 in *Physiology* 3rd ed.)

8. Hypokalemia prevents generation of normal neuronal action potentials, and thus impairs neuro-muscular function. In the heart, repolarization is primarily affected, so that on the electrocardiogram, T-waves are flat or disappear entirely, and a late U-wave is generated. (See p. 374 in *Physiology* 3rd ed.)

9. Although extracellular fluid volume is expanded modestly by an excess of aldosterone, escape from a continuous positive sodium balance with gross edema occurs by two mechanisms. Glomerular filtration rate is increased, and with it the filtered load of sodium, so that a greater percentage of filtered sodium escapes reabsorption. The expanded extracellular fluid volume also stimulates secretion of atrial natriuretic hormone, which offsets the effect of aldosterone by directly inhibiting sodium reabsorption in the collecting ducts. (See pp. 774-775 in *Physiology* 3rd ed.)

10. Normal secretion of insulin in response to glucose depends on normal extracellular potassium concentrations. Hypokalemia decreases pancreatic islet beta cell function and therefore fasting plasma glucose may increase. (See p. 859 in *Physiology* 3rd ed.)

11. The patient probably has primary hyperaldosteronism, that is, autonomous hypersecretion from an adenoma of the adrenal zona glomerulosa. Therefore levels of renin and generation of angiotensin I will be reduced. The patient's hypertension will not be very dependent on conversion of angiotensin I to angiotensin II, which is the powerful vasoconstrictor. Therefore converting enzyme inhibitor therapy was not very effective. (See p. 966 in *Physiology* 3rd ed.)

12. The logical treatment was the administration of an aldosterone antagonist. By binding to and blocking the aldosterone receptor, renal tubular sodium reabsorption and potassium secretion would be decreased, which would allow plasma potassium to rise to normal and blood pressure to fall to normal. (See pp. 968 and 969 in *Physiology* 3rd ed.)

Case 2

1. The constellation of signs and symptoms in this patient is a classic picture of the effects of excess cortisol or of any exogenously administered glucocorticoid. (See pp. 959-964 in *Physiology* 3rd ed.)

2. Cortisol creates an antianabolic (i.e., catabolic) metabolic state. The muscle mass shows increased proteolysis with a resulting decrease in the size and number of muscle fibers and consequently by weakness and atrophy. In bone, collagen synthesis is inhibited and the rate of bone resorption is increased, which leads to osteopenia and to fractures. Calcium absorption from the gastrointestinal tract is diminished because of inhibition of the action of 1,25-$(OH)_2$ vitamin D. This adds to the difficulty in maintaining bone mass. Inhibition of collagen synthesis in skin and blood vessel walls leads to thinning of these tissues and to fragility of capillaries; this causes bruising and purple bands in the skin. Appetite is stimulated centrally by cortisol, but the excess of ingested calories is selectively deposited in certain depots for reasons currently unexplained. Cortisol decreases REM sleep and increases the amount of time awake. All of the above effects stem from the binding of cortisol to its nuclear glucocorticoid receptor (type II). This modulates the transcription of numerous genes. (See pp. 884 and 958-964 in *Physiology* 3rd ed.)

3. Cortisol inhibits the insulin-stimulated uptake of glucose by muscle and augments gluconeogenesis in the liver. These effects combine to raise fasting plasma glucose. Plasma insulin increases in response to the rise in plasma glucose. (See pp. 858-860, 962, and 963 in *Physiology* 3rd ed.)

4. Cortisol also binds to the mineralocorticoid receptor (type I glucocorticoid receptor), and an excess of cortisol can therefore mimic aldosterone actions on the kidney to produce sodium retention, edema, hypertension, hypokalemia, and metabolic alkalosis. (See pp. 959 and 968-969 in *Physiology* 3rd ed.)

5. Cortisol has marked effects on the hematopoietic system. Recruitment of neutrophils from the bone marrow is stimulated, but their margination and transfer to tissue are inhibited so that the circulating number rises. Lymphocyte numbers decrease. (See pp. 964-965 in *Physiology* 3rd ed.)

6. Hypersecretion of cortisol would be established by one or more of the following findings. The plasma cortisol level would be elevated in the morning but especially in the evening (a time of day when plasma cortisol normally is low because of diurnal variation). A 24-hour urinary excretion of free cortisol would be elevated. A 24-hour urinary excretion of metabolites of cortisol (17-hydroxy corticoids) would also be elevated when corrected for body mass or when expressed per gram of creatinine. (See pp. 955-958 in *Physiology* 3rd ed.)

7. Hypersecretion of cortisol could result from abnormalities at various points in the hypothalamic-pituitary adrenal axis.

    a. A benign or malignant adrenal neoplasm may secrete excess cortisol.

    b. Increased secretion of ACTH by a pituitary neoplasm or in response to an excess of corticotropin-releasing hormone may stimulate excess secretion of cortisol by both adrenal glands (adrenal hyperplasia). ACTH may also be secreted by nonpituitary neoplasms that express the propio-melanocortin gene. (See pp. 905-906 in *Physiology* 3rd ed.)

8.   a. Autonomous hypersecretion of cortisol by an adrenal neoplasm should suppress ACTH secretion by negative feedback. Hence plasma ACTH level will be low. (See pp. 906-908 in *Physiology* 3rd ed.)

    b. If hypersecretion of cortisol is caused by a pituitary lesion, plasma ACTH will be elevated or at least inappropriately normal in the face of elevated cortisol levels. This resetting of the normal relationship between cortisol and ACTH can be demonstrated by administering an appropriate dose of a synthetic glucocorticoid, such as dexamethasone. In a normal individual, this will markedly decrease both plasma ACTH and plasma cortisol levels, but in an individual with abnormally functioning pituitary corticotrophs, plasma ACTH and cortisol will decrease little, if any. However, if a very large dose of dexamethasone is given, even the abnormal corticotrophs will be shut off, and plasma ACTH and cortisol will decrease significantly. (See pp. 906-908 in *Physiology* 3rd ed.)

    c.   Abnormal expression of the ACTH precursor gene by a nonendocrine tumor will be manifest by a very high plasma level of ACTH, with no suppression when dexamethasone is given. In addition, such high levels of ACTH may cause hyperpigmentation of the skin because of the melanocyte-stimulating hormone sequence within ACTH. (See pp. 905-906 in *Physiology* 3rd ed.)

9.   The loss of regular menses and the increasing facial hair suggest an excess of adrenal androgen secretion. Plasma levels of dehydroepiandrosterone and androstenedione will likely be elevated. These weak androgens may then be converted to the potent androgen, testosterone, in peripheral tissues. (See pp. 953, 966, and 986 in *Physiology* 3rd ed.)

10.   This patient's hypercortisolism was found to be caused by an adrenal adenoma. Therefore her plasma ACTH level was very low because of negative feedback. As a result, the remaining normal adrenal cortical tissue was atrophic and nonfunctioning. Immediately after removal of the adrenal adenoma, the plasma cortisol fell to low levels, which produced her postoperative symptoms and low blood pressure. This situation can persist for many months until, first, her adrenocorticotrophs recover from prolonged suppression and, second, her remaining adrenal cortical cells increase in size and number and recover their ability to secrete normal amounts of cortisol. (See p. 963 in *Physiology* 3rd ed.)

CHAPTER 51

Case 1

1. This individual could have an XX karyotype. The blind ending to the vagina and absence of the uterus could be explained by failure of embryologic development of the Mullerian ducts bilaterally. However, this would not explain the presence of apparent gonads in the inguinal canals, nor would it explain the absence of sexual hair, which implies deficient androgenic stimulation. (See pp. 966 and 982 in *Physiology* 3rd ed.)

2. It is highly unlikely that this individual has an XO karyotype. It is true that such a karyotype would allow feminization of the external genitalia, because this process requires only the absence of androgen activity. However, Mullerian duct development would still occur normally, because without a Y chromosome there is no production of anti-Mullerian hormone. Therefore a uterus and cervix should have been detected on physical examination. Furthermore, in subjects in the XO state, the ovaries do not function; therefore little or no estrogen secretion or breast development occurs. Finally, the patient's height is normal, whereas XO individuals are usually short. (See pp. 981, 983, and 984 in *Physiology* 3rd ed.)

3. This individual certainly could have an XY chromosome karyotype. If she were XY, the completely female external genitalia suggests an absence of androgenic activity, because androgens are required to masculinize the external genitalia in a normal male. The lack of sexual hair confirms the absence of androgenic activity. The lack of androgen could be accounted for by a defect in the synthesis of testosterone, by deficient production of dihydrotestosterone from testosterone because of deficiency of the enzyme 5 α-reductase, or by the lack of an androgen receptor. (See pp. 981-983 and 986 in *Physiology* 3rd ed.)

    Defects in testosterone synthesis are usually partial and do not produce absolute androgen deficiency. Therefore Wolffian duct development occurs, and external genitalia are ambiguous rather than completely feminine. A lack of testosterone would also not account for the breast development, because the breasts are estrogen dependent and androgens are a necessary precursor to estrogen synthesis. Dihydrotestosterone is required for in utero masculinization of the external genitalia (though not for Wolffian duct development). Hence, dihydrotestosterone deficiency could account for the feminine pattern. However, during puberty, testosterone itself, without conversion to dihydrotestosterone, can stimulate growth of the penis; but this obviously did not occur in the patient. Dihydrotestosterone deficiency would also not induce marked breast development, because normal testosterone levels would still balance normal estrogen levels and inhibit breast development in an XY individual. Absence of the androgen receptor would explain all of the patient's findings. Without tissue receptors, testosterone could not promote Wolffian duct development, and dihydrotestosterone could not masculinize the external genitalia. The growth of sexual hair could not be stimulated. Lack of androgen receptor in the breast tissue would also allow unopposed estrogen action and therefore good or even excessive breast development. (See pp. 981, 983-986, 1000, and 1001 in *Physiology* 3rd ed.)

4. The inguinal masses in this XY individual would be testes, because differentiation of the indifferent gonads into testes requires materials from the Y chromosome. The spermatogenic apparatus would be poorly developed, however, because of the lack of essential local testosterone action on Sertoli cells and possibly on the germ cells themselves. The Leydig cells would be hyperplastic, reflecting high rates of testosterone production. This would compensate for resistance to the testosterone action

caused by androgen receptor deficiency. (See pp. 980-982, 985, 986, and 994-996 in *Physiology* 3rd ed.)

5.   For this XY individual, the plasma LH level would be elevated because of loss of negative feedback by testosterone on the pituitary gonadotrophs, which would also lack the androgen receptor. The high LH levels would stimulate increased secretion of testosterone by the hyperplastic Leydig cells. In turn, high testosterone levels would lead to overproduction of estradiol by the testes and also by peripheral conversion. The plasma level of FSH would be normal because of normal production of inhibin by the Sertoli cells.

    If this were an XX individual with failure of Mullerian duct development, the levels of testosterone, estradiol, LH, and FSH in the plasma would all be normal.

    In an XO individual, plasma estradiol would be low because granulosa cell function is absent. Plasma testosterone might also be low because of a lack of theca cell function. Plasma LH would be high because of a lack of negative feedback by estradiol. Plasma FSH would be high because of a lack of inhibin production caused by absence of granulosa cells. (See pp. 913, 985, 986, 994, and 1003-1008 in *Physiology* 3rd ed.)

Case 2

1.   a.   Although apparently normal, the husband's sperm could fail to undergo capacitation in the patient's vaginal tract. (See pp. 993-994 in *Physiology* 3rd ed.)

        b.   The husband's sperm could be rejected by the patient's ova during attempted fertilization (e.g., because of antisperm antibodies). (See pp. 1014-1015 in *Physiology* 3rd ed.)

        c.   Though the patient does menstruate, she might not recruit and develop a dominant follicle. (See pp. 1006-1008 in *Physiology* 3rd ed.)

        d.   The dominant follicle might not receive the proper signal to undergo ovulation. (See pp. 1004 and 1008 in *Physiology* 3rd ed.)

        e.   An ovulated egg might not be picked up by a diseased ipsilateral fallopian tube, or such a tube might not allow ascent of sperm or descent of a fertilized egg. (See p. 1014 in *Physiology* 3rd ed.)

        f.   A corpus luteum might fail to form or function normally. This failure would result in inadequate nourishment of a fertilized ovum or inadequate preparation of an implantation site for the zygote. (See pp. 1003-1004, 1008, and 1016 in *Physiology* 3rd ed.)

        g.   Secure implantation might never occur because of local uterine abnormalities, and thus the patient was having clinically undetected abortions. (See p. 1015 in *Physiology* 3rd ed.)

2.   a.   The husband's sperm could be recovered from the vaginal tract after intercourse and examined to determine its motility. Its ability to penetrate an ovum could be determined in vitro by interacting it with a test receptive ovum, such as from a hamster. (See pp. 993 and 1014 in *Physiology* 3rd ed.)

b. The husband's sperm could be reacted in vitro with eggs retrieved from the wife after ovulation. The presence of antibodies to sperm could be sought on the patient's ova or in her serum. Both sperm and ova could be washed to eliminate such putative antibodies before allowing them to interact.

c. The pattern of plasma estradiol changes during the patient's menstrual cycle would be examined. Failure to develop a dominant follicle would be reflected by the absence of an accelerated rise in plasma estradiol during the presumptive late follicular phase of the cycle. This failure in turn might be due to a low plasma FSH level in the early follicular phase of the cycle or a low plasma LH level in the midfollicular phase of the cycle. Inadequate secretion of FSH and LH could be caused by intrinsic pituitary diseases or by a hypothalamic disorder.

A demonstration that LH and FSH levels increase normally after administration of gonadotropin-releasing hormone (GnRH) would incriminate a lack of normal GnRH secretion rather than a pituitary abnormality. Such hypothalamic reproductive dysfunction could be caused by stress, excessive exercise, or eating disorders. A high plasma prolactin level would indicate hypersecretion of prolactin, which inhibits GnRH release. Alternatively, failure to develop a dominant follicle could be caused by intrinsic resistance of granulosa or theca cells, for example, because of deficiency of LH and/or FSH receptors. In this case, plasma LH and FSH levels would be high. (See pp. 911, 912, 923, 1004, and 1009 in *Physiology* 3rd ed.)

d. Failure to observe a midcycle surge in plasma or urine LH and FSH would indicate lack of generation of a normal ovulatory signal. Entrapped dominant follicles degenerate into cysts, which can be visualized by ultrasound examination of the ovaries. (See pp. 914, 1004, and 1009 in *Physiology* 3rd ed.)

e. Blockage of the fallopian tubes can be demonstrated by injection of x-ray dye into the uterus, with failure of the dye to reach the peritoneal cavity.

f. A failure of corpus luteum function would be indicated by a lack of the normal rise in plasma progesterone during the presumptive luteal phase of the cycle. It would also be reflected histologically by the absence of a secretory pattern of the endometrium on biopsy and by persistence of estrogen-stimulated vaginal mucosal cells and cervical mucus patterns. (See pp. 1004 and 1009-1011 in *Physiology* 3rd ed.)

g. Detection of a transient rise in the plasma level of human chorionic gonadotropin late in the patient's menstrual cycle would indicate that conception had occurred, but that the zygotes were being aborted after unsuccessful implantation and were being passed with the menstrual slough. (See pp. 1011 and 1015 in *Physiology* 3rd ed.)

3. a. Direct insertion of the husband's washed sperm into the uterus (i.e., artificial insemination) could be used to bypass inadequate capacitation in the vaginal tract. Alternatively, in vitro fertilization could be carried out with the husband's sperm and the patient's retrieved ova.

b. A failure of normal follicular development could be treated by stimulation of hypothalamic GnRH releases with appropriate drugs. Alternatively, exogenous GnRH could be administered in pulsatile fashion to elicit a normal pattern of gonadotropin secretion and normal follicular development. The entire hypothalamic pituitary part of the axis could be bypassed by administering FSH and LH daily in appropriate doses and then supplying a large LH dose to elicit ovulation at the appropriate time indicated by the plasma estradiol level. The latter treatment would be appropriate in the answer to 2d. (See pp. 912, 1004, 1008, and 1012 in *Physiology* 3rd ed.)

c. Blockage of fallopian tubes can be bypassed by in vitro fertilization after retrieval of the patient's ova from the peritoneal cavity.

d. Administration of progesterone during the latter half of the cycle would replace inadequate function of the corpus luteum. (See pp. 1004 and 1016 in *Physiology* 3rd ed.)

e. Failure of implantation mechanisms could be treated by using the retrieved ova of the patient and her husband's sperm for in vitro fertilization. The resultant fertilized eggs could be implanted in the uterus of a surrogate mother of proven fertility. (See pp. 1009-1010 in *Physiology* 3rd ed.)